"An interesting and useful collection of essays on three seemingly chronic, tenacious, and coupled problems— cocaine dependence, injecting drug use, and AIDS. The authors, all very well-known in their fields, have applied their knowledge and years of experience to each of these challenges, exploring a variety of approaches for the management of cocaine withdrawal and relapse. In addition and especially important, are the variety of insights offered in the papers addressing AIDS-risk reduction initiatives for injecting drug users and their sex partners. A... significant contribution to our understanding of the AIDS/IV drug connection and the mechanisms for dealing with it."

—James A. Inciardi, PhD, Professor and Director, Center for Drug and Alcohol Studies, University of Delaware

D0967317

Cocaine, AIDS, and Intravenous Drug Use

Cocaine, AIDS, and Intravenous Drug Use

Samuel R. Friedman, PhD
Douglas S. Lipton, PhD
Guest Editors

Barry Stimmel, MD
Editor

Cocaine, AIDS, and Intravenous Drug Use, edited by Barry Stimmel, Samuel R. Friedman and Douglas S. Lipton, was simultaneously issued by The Haworth Press, Inc., under the same title, as a special issue of the *Journal of Addictive Diseases,* Volume 10, Number 4 1991, Barry Stimmel, Editor.

Harrington Park Press
An Imprint of The Haworth Press, Inc.
New York • London • Sydney

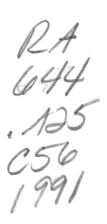

ISBN 1-56023-004-5

Published by

Harrington Park Press, 10 Alice Street, Binghamton, NY 13904-1580
EUROSPAN/Harrington, 3 Henrietta Street, London WC2E 8LU England
ASTAM/Harrington, 162-168 Parramatta Road, Stanmore, Sydney, N.S.W. 2048 Australia

Harrington Park Press is an imprint of The Haworth Press, Inc., 10 Alice Street, Binghamton, NY 13904-1580

Cocaine, AIDS, and Intravenous Drug Use was originally published as *Journal of Addictive Diseases,* Volume 10, Number 4 1991.

Library of Congress Cataloging-in-Publication Data

Cocaine, AIDS, and intravenous drug use / Samuel R. Friedman, / Douglas S. Lipton, Barry Stimmel, editors.
    p. cm.
    "Simultaneously issued by The Haworth Press, Inc. . . . as special issue of the Journal of addictive diseases, volume 10, number 4, 1991."
    Includes bibliographical references (p.).
    ISBN 1-56023-004-5 (acid-free paper) (HPP)
    1. AIDS (Disease) – Prevention. 2. Cocaine habit. 3. Intravenous drug abuse. I. Friedman, Samuel R., 1942- . II Lipton, Douglas S. III. Stimmel, Barry, 1939 .
    RA644.A25C56 1991b
    616.97'9205 – dc20   91-27471
                                                      CIP

Cocaine, AIDS, and Intravenous Drug Use

CONTENTS

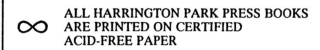

ABOUT THE GUEST EDITORS

Samuel R. Friedman, PhD, is Principal Investigator on a number of research projects to develop and assess ways to assist IV drug users and their sexual partners reduce their risks of becoming infected with or passing HIV to others. He has written more than fifty publications on AIDS and IV drug use. He is a member of the Steering Committees of the International Working Group on AIDS Among Intravenous Drug Users and the Sociology AIDS Network and has consulted for the Centers for Disease Control and the World Health Organization.

Douglas S. Lipton, PhD, has served as Director of Research and a member of the Board of Directors for NDRI, as well as Deputy Director of the New York Division of Substance Abuse Services in charge of state drug abuse research. He has evaluated drug abuse control and treatment programs around the world for the United Nations.

EDITORIAL

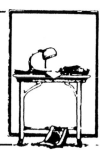

Cocaine, AIDS and IV Drug Use

Cocaine use and AIDS have become over the last decade two issues of great concern not only to the public but also to those engaged in the field of substance abuse. In the third week of October, 1989, more than 700 professionals, service providers and policy makers gathered in New York City to present and listen to the most current research information in the field of drug use. This international conference, attended by persons from five continents, was co-sponsored by the New York State Division of Substance Abuse Services and by Narcotic and Drug Research, Inc., a New York City-based non-profit research and training institute established in 1967. The focus of the gathering was to: (1) present in lay language what works and what doesn't work; (2) present new methods being tested; and (3) generate a research agenda for the 1990s. A number of the papers included in this volume emerged from this conference.

1

COCAINE

NIDA, in 1984, declared cocaine the drug of greatest national health concern. Notwithstanding that the "cocaine epidemic" and "crack plague" have been the subjects of media hyperbole since the mid-eighties, peaking in the 1987-1988 period,[1] there has been a genuine increase in the numbers and severity of the casualties to cocaine in its various forms. Explorations into psychosocial approaches and pharmacologic approaches thus have been urged, and although treatment has frequently met with frustrating outcomes, the beginnings of breakthroughs can be seen. Crosby, Halikas and Carlson[2] deal with psychopharmacologic agents in the therapeutic management of the cocaine addict's physical and psychological withdrawal symptoms. Of particular note is their paper's organization of pharmacologic agents by current hypotheses of neurotransmitter function and cocaine dependency: (a) dopamine depletion with agents like bromocriptine and amantadine, (b) receptor supersensitivity with agents like tricyclic antidepressants, (c) direct symptom relief with benzodiazepines and neuroleptics, (d) cocaine-induced kindling with agents like carbamazepine, and (e) serotonin antagonist with agents like L-tryptophan, fluvoxamine and fluoxetine.

The relapse of formerly stable methadone patients to cocaine use is a distressing consequence of the growth of cocaine use generally. While methadone lessens or eliminates heroin's effects, methadone may have the opposite effect when used simultaneously with cocaine, akin to experiencing a "speedball." Rates of cocaine use among methadone patients are reported to be as high as 70%,[3,4] but generally in the forty to fifty percent range.[5,6] The article by Magura et al. examines a sample of methadone patients admitted to four clinics during 1987, 84 percent of whom were cocaine users at entry.[7] It reports the changes that occurred in their program status, cocaine use, and heroin use as well as their injecting behaviors after remaining in treatment for varying lengths of time, and suggest a new perspective for a remedy. Realistic consideration of treatment for cocaine users must consider that the bulk of cocaine users also use other substances, notably alcohol.[8] The sequelae to the nervous system and other systems of the combined use of cocaine and alcohol have not been examined very frequently.[9,10] Moskowitz, Errichetti and colleagues have compared the effects of long term alcohol and chronic cocaine-alcohol exposure on cardiac function with some interesting findings relevant to treatment.[11]

AIDS AND DRUG USERS

Four of the articles in this volume deal with how to prevent the further spread of the AIDS epidemic. This is not a pleasant topic to have to deal with, and it can lead treatment programs and agencies into activities that may upset their previous assumptions. It is important to start from a realistic understanding of the choices we face. A list of some hard realities will set a useful framework:

1. Drug injection will not be stopped by police action or other forms of drug interdiction. At most, these will reduce supplies and deter some persons from beginning to use drugs.
2. Drug prevention programs may reduce recruitment of new drug users, but will not stop it altogether. Further, there are already hundreds of thousands of drug injectors in the United States who will remain as a pool of people who can become infected with HIV.
3. There are far fewer slots in drug abuse treatment programs than there are drug injectors. If we add in those smokers, sniffers, and snorters who are at high risk of becoming injectors, the lack of treatment capacity becomes even clearer. Further, it is often the drug injectors who are least able to contribute financially to their treatment.
4. Drug abuse treatment saves thousands of persons from addiction, but many who complete their treatment relapse to drug use.
5. Many users who enter treatment either continue to inject while being treated, drop out of treatment, or are expelled from treatment.
6. Many drug injectors do not want to enter treatment. Others may want only partial treatment.
7. Attempts to stigmatize or repress drug users can drive them further underground. This can make it harder for non-users to

screen potential sex partners for prior or current risks (and thus increase heterosexual transmission of HIV). It can also reduce the social ties between drug injectors and their non-injector friends and relatives; but there is some evidence that these ties are protective in that drug injectors who retain them are more likely to take more precautions against becoming infected.[12]

8. HIV can spread rapidly, but need not do so. In the course of one year, almost half of the drug injectors in Bangkok, Thailand, became infected. In New York City, southern Manhattan seropositivity rates increased from 9% to over 40% in two years. Yet in San Francisco, seropositivity has remained in the 10% to 20% range for several years.[13,14]

On the positive side, many drug injectors have already taken steps to reduce their own risks and those of others,[15] and seroprevalence has stabilized in a number of cities.[13,14] Further, many projects have been set up to encourage further risk reduction. A number of articles in this volume discuss risk reduction projects.

Reaching Drug Injectors

The article by Sorensen reviews AIDS risk reduction in drug treatment programs.[16] He bases both his own risk reduction projects and his discussion in this paper around the Health Belief Model (HBM). The HBM argues that risk reducing changes are the result of appropriate health beliefs, namely (1) a perceived threat, in that drug injectors come to believe that AIDS threatens them; (2) perceived benefits, in that they come to believe there are ways for them to protect themselves; (3) self-efficacy, in that they believe that they have the ability to perform the actions needed to protect themselves; and (4) social support, in that others support them in their efforts to reduce their risk. He then discusses a number of projects that use small group interventions, individual counseling, and/or antibody testing and counseling, to promote risk reduction. On the basis of studies that show some success in these efforts, he argues that what is needed now is to consolidate these studies in an attempt to take the most successful elements of each and find ways to combine them into optimally effective interventions. Such techniques then need to be disseminated to treatment programs in ways that will get them accepted. Since relatively few clients have eliminated their high risk behavior completely, however, and since even risk reduction is often difficult to sustain over a period of several years, we are skeptical of Sorensen's argument that the essential outlines of risk reduction projects are known and thus of his advocacy of incremental improvement rather than combining this with the testing of altogether new models.

The papers by Hagan et al. and Sufian et al. both discuss interventions that promulgate risk reduction among drug injectors who are accessed in non-treatment settings.[17,18] In both cases, one of the goals of the intervention is to encourage the users to enter drug abuse treatment, but this is seen as only one of several important risk reduction approaches.

Hagan views syringe exchanges as having several useful effects. Most obviously, they provide drug injectors with sterile injection equipment, thus providing them with the means to protect themselves against HIV, as well as removing potentially infected syringes from the streets. They also provide a setting in which staff and drug injectors interact, allowing health education, referrals, and the distribution of other useful items.

Hagan reports that participants in the syringe exchange reduce a wide range of risk behaviors. Although clients continue to inject at about the same frequency, there is no evidence that they have increased their drug use. Nor is there any evidence that the program has led anyone to be recruited into drug injection. These findings, it should be added, broadly parallel those of evaluations of the Dutch,[19,20] British,[14] and Australian[21,22] syringe exchange schemes.

Syringe exchanges of the type discussed by Hagan et al. have been quite controversial in the United States, but have been much less so in the Netherlands, England, and Australia. Indeed, many Europeans look aghast upon American reluctance to implement such programs, seeing it as akin to failing to provide life preservers to someone who is drowning. The syringe exchange in Tacoma that is the subject of this paper was the first exchange in the United States, and came into existence by the informal action of one man with considerable experience working with drug users. This reflects the fact that there have been three different forms of syringe exchanges — informal, semi-legal ones such as that in Tacoma or such as the first ones that were set up by Dutch drug users' unions in the early 1980s; formal programs endorsed by government agencies such as most of those in the United Kingdom, the Netherlands, and Washington State today; and illegal, underground exchanges such as those in many New England cities, New York City, and San Francisco. The formal programs have probably been most effective in distributing large numbers of syringes, but it remains to be seen whether the underground and/or informal exchanges might be particularly effective in producing risk reduction by virtue of the solidarity produced between volunteer staff members and the drug injectors with whom they work.

Sufian et al. report on a project that attempted to organize drug injectors against AIDS. This project was developed with an eye to the successful organizations gay men have set up to promote risk education and, indeed, to wage a war within their subcultures to create norms, values, interests, and institutions conducive to low risk activities. It also drew upon observations of the successes and problems of the Dutch drug users' unions (*junkiebonden*) and their efforts against AIDS.[23,15] Since it began, a second effort to organize drug users against AIDS was started in Minneapolis-St. Paul.[24]

The project reported on by Sufian had a number of difficulties in implementation—which was to be expected in the first project of its kind. On the other hand, the impact evaluation of the project reports considerable risk reduction. The data on follow-up are given somewhat more of a context by comparing them to those reported by projects in Chicago, Houston, Miami, Philadelphia, and San Francisco in a recent article in the *Mortality and Morbidity Weekly Report*.[25] Subjects in the organizing projects were considerably more likely to report always using condoms during sex (33% vs. 25% in Miami and less in the other four cities) and entry into drug abuse treatment (47% vs. 35% in San Francisco and less in the other four cities). On the other hand, the 19% who always used bleach in the organizing project was much less than the 43% reported for San Francisco but similar to figures reported for the other cities. Bleach use has been the major emphasis of outreach projects in San Francisco (which have been able to field 50-100 outreach workers for 20,000 drug injectors, as compared to approximately 50 outreach workers in all of New York City to reach 200,000 drug injectors).

In sum, then, the project Sufian reports on shows considerable promise. Further research on projects to organize drug users against AIDS seems warranted.

Female Sex Partners and HIV Infection

Cohen's article is an excellent and deeply moving review of what is known about the HIV-related problems faced by women who do not inject drugs but who have drug injecting sex partners.[26] She discusses the extent of heterosexual transmission of the virus and the difficulties of reaching women whose defining common characteristic is drug injection by their sex partners. A large proportion of these women share other characteristics: many face economic need, many are members of racially oppressed groups, many have a wide variety of unmet medical needs, and many are deeply involved in (non-injected) drug use. Cohen despairs at the likelihood of getting male drug injectors to use condoms; data such as those presented by Sufian et al., if validated, may indicate that some drug injectors can come to consistently use condoms, but even Sufian's data indicate consistent condom use by only one drug injector in three.

Cohen emphasizes the *process* by which information is made available to female partners as being at least as important as its content. Locating the female partners has also been problematic — usually, drug abuse treatment and AIDS-related programs have been less effective than sessions held at less stigmatized locations. She also discusses the difficult dilemmas faced by women who learn they are actually or potentially infected through their partner's or child's being diagnosed as infected with HIV, and discusses the problems these issues pose both for the women and for antibody testing programs.

One limitation of Cohen's article should be pointed out. She sees sex partners primarily as "clients," i.e., as people to be brought to projects where they will be educated and perhaps empowered. We would like to suggest that a community organizing model might also be useful. Here, two diagrams might be helpful in explaining what we mean. Figure 1 presents the client-oriented, agency-centered model. The active agent is the agency or peer group; it communicates with the woman partner, who is left alone to deal with her relationships with her drug injecting male partner and anyone else she chooses.

A community organizing model is presented in Figure 2. Here, the organizing agency attempts to bring both members of the couple, and their friends and relatives, into the process. It does this by working within the community as a whole, as well as with specific persons involved, to change norms, values and practices that bear

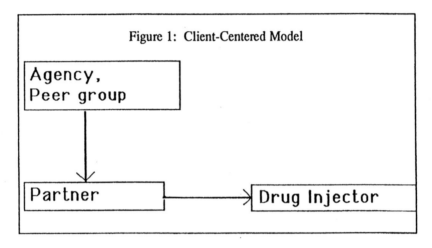

Figure 1: Client-Centered Model

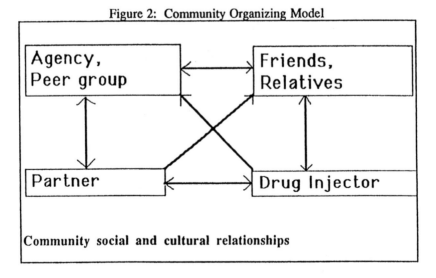

Figure 2: Community Organizing Model

on condom use and partnerships. Thus, it aims to legitimate condom use; to repudiate opposition to condom use; and to create a supportive environment for the peaceful and successful resolution of disputes over sexual risk taking. Attempts are in progress to develop this model.

SUMMARY

The papers in this volume cover a wide range of important topics. Yet many other equally important topics are not addressed. These include: (1) emerging trends in the epidemiology of HIV and drug use, such as the evidence that crack use may lead many of its practitioners to engage in high risk sex; (2) ways to deliver HIV prophylaxis to infected drug injectors, sexual partners, or perinatally infected children; and (3) the effectiveness of standard outreach in encouraging risk reduction. They do, however, provide important information about how to deal with both cocaine use and AIDS. They also raise many fruitful issues for additional research.

We are grateful to Susan Weiman and wish to acknowledge her for her special editorial assistance.

Samuel R. Friedman
Douglas S. Lipton

REFERENCES

1. Reinarman, C. & Levine, H.G. Crack in context: Politics and media in the making of a drug scare. *Contemporary Drug Problems* 1989; 17: 535-578.

2. Crosby, R.D., Halikas, J.A., Carlson, G. Pharmacotherapeutic interventions for cocaine abuse: Present practices and future directions. *Journal of Addictive Diseases* 1991 10: 13-30.

3. Kosten, T.R., Gawin, F.H., Rounsaville, B.J. & Kleber, H.D. Cocaine abuse among opioid addicts: Demographic and diagnostic factors in treatment. *American J. Drug & Alcohol Abuse* 1986; 12:1-16.

4. Kosten, T.R., Rounsaville, B.J. & Kleber H.D. A 2.5 year follow up of cocaine use among treated opioid addicts: Have our treatments helped? *Arch General Psychiatry* 1987; 44: 281-284.

5. Black, J.L., Dolan, M.P., Penk, W.E., Robinowitz, R. & DeFord, H.A. The effect of increased cocaine use on drug treatment. *Addictive Behaviors* 1987, 12: 289-292.

6. Hartel, D., Schoenbaum, E.E., Selwyn, P.A., Drucker, E., Wasserman, W. & Friedland, G.W. Temporal patterns of cocaine use and AIDS in intravenous drug users in methadone maintenance. Presented at the Fifth International Conference on AIDS, Montreal, Canada, 1989.

7. Magura, S., Siddiqi, Q., Freeman, R.C., Lipton, D.S. Changes in cocaine use after entry to methadone treatment. *Journal of Addictive Diseases* 1991: 10: 31-45.

8. Smith, D.E. Cocaine-alcohol abuse: Epidemiological, diagnostic and treatment considerations. *J. Psychoactive Drugs* 1986; 18: 117-29.

9. St. John, A., Vullilet, P.R. & Avakian, E.V. Effects of chronic cocaine administration on rat cardiac and splenic norepinephrine levels. *Proc. Western Pharmacology Society* 1989; 32: 61-63.

10. Wiener, R.S., Lockhart, J.T., & Schwartz, R.G. Dilated cardiomyopathy and cocaine abuse. Report of two cases. *American J. Medicine* 1986; 81: 699-701.

11. Moskowitz, R.M. & Errichetti, A.J. Cardiovascular evaluation after withdrawal from chronic alcohol or cocaine-alcohol abuse. *Journal of Addictive Diseases* 1991; 10: 47-65.

12. Neaigus A., Friedman, S.R., Sufian M. et al. Social contact and risk reduction among IV users. Presented at APHA, N.Y.C. 1990.

13. Des Jarlais, D.C., Friedman, S.R., Novick, D.M., Sotheran, J.L., Thomas, P., Yancovitz, S.R., Mildvan, D., Weber, J., Kreck, M.J., Maslansky, R., Spira, T., Marmor, M. HIV-1 Infection among intravenous drug users in Manhattan, New York City, from 1977 through 1987. *JAMA* 261 (Feb. 17, 1989) 7:1008-1012.

14. Stimson, G.V. Preventing spread of HIV in injecting drug users: Current advances and remaining obstacles. Presented at the Sixth International AIDS Conference, San Francisco, 1990 (forthcoming, *British J. Addictions*).

15. Friedman, S.R., Des Jarlais, D.C., Sotheran, J.L., Garber, J., Cohen, H., Smith, D. AIDS and self-organization among intravenous drug users. *International J. Addictions* 1987; 22(3): 201-219.

16. Sorenson, J.L. Preventing HIV transmission in drug treatment programs: What works? *Journal of Addictive Diseases* 1991. 10: 67-79.

17. Hagan, H., Des Jarlais, D.C., Purchase, D., Reid, T., & Friedman, S.R. The Tacoma syringe exchange. *Journal of Addictive Diseases* 1991. 10: 81-88.

18. Sufian, M., Friedman, S.R., Curtis, R., Neaigus, A. & Stepherson, B. Organizing as a new approach to AIDS risk reduction for intravenous drug users. *Journal of Addictive Diseases* 1991. 10: 89-98.

19. Buning, E.C., van Brussel, G.H.A., van Santen, G. Amsterdam's drug policy and its implications for controlling needle sharing. In Battjes, R.J. and Pickens, R.W. eds, *Needle Sharing among Intravenous Drug Abusers: National and International Perspectives*. (NIDA Research Monograph 80) Washington, DC: US GPO, 1988, 59-74.

20. van den Hoek, J.A.R., van Haastrecht, H.J.A., & Coutinho, R.A. Risk

reduction among intravenous drug users in Amsterdam under the influence of AIDS. *American J. Public Health*, 1989; 79: 1355-1357.

21. Stimson, G.V. Syringe-exchanges programmes for injecting drug users. *AIDS* 1989; 3: 253-260.

22. Wodak, A., Dolan, K., Imrie, A.A., Gold, J., Wolk, J., Whyte, B.M., & Cooper, D.A. Antibodies to the human immunodeficiency virus in needles and syringes used by intravenous drug abusers. *Medical J. Australia* 1987; 147: 275-276. 1987.

23. Friedman, S.R., de Jong, W.M., Des Jarlais, D.C. Problems and dynamics of organizing intravenous drug users for AIDS prevention. *Health Education Research*. 1988; 3:49-57.

24. Carlson, G. & Needle, R. Sponsoring addict self-organization (Addicts Against AIDS): A case study. 1st Annual National AIDS Demonstration Research Conference, Rockville, MD. 1989.

25. Centers for Disease Control. Update: Reducing HIV transmission in intravenous drug users not in drug treatment—United States. *MMWR* 39;31 (August 10, 1990): 529, 535-539.

26. Cohen, J.B. Why women partners of drug users will continue to be at high risk for HIV infection. *Journal of Addictive Diseases* 1991 10: 99-110.

Pharmacotherapeutic Interventions for Cocaine Abuse: Present Practices and Future Directions

Ross D. Crosby, PhD
James A. Halikas, MD
Gregory Carlson, BA

SUMMARY. The therapeutic management of the cocaine addict deals with a wide range of physical and psychological withdrawal symptoms, including a sometimes overwhelming craving for cocaine. Many medications have been used in the treatment of cocaine withdrawal and dependence, using as a rationale, known pharmacologic effects of cocaine on neurotransmitters. Animal observations related to dopamine depletion, receptor supersensitivity, cocaine-induced kindling, and serotonin depletion have all generated pharmacotherapeutic interventions for cocaine abuse. An extensive review of the use of these agents is presented. Pharmacotherapeutic strategies in dealing with the methadone-maintained cocaine abuser are considered. Future areas of interest and limitations of pharmacotherapy in dealing with cocaine abuse are discussed.

Ross D. Crosby is Assistant Research Professor, Department of Psychiatry, University of Minnesota; James A. Halikas is Professor of Psychiatry, University of Minnesota School of Medicine, and Director, Chemical Dependency Treatment Program, University of Minnesota Hospital and Clinic; and Gregory Carlson is Administrative Director, Department of Psychiatry, Chemical Dependency Treatment Program, University of Minnesota.

Address requests and correspondence to Ross D. Crosby, PhD, Department of Psychiatry, Box 393 Mayo, University of Minnesota, 420 Delaware Street, Minneapolis, MN 55455.

INTRODUCTION

The increase in cocaine use during the last decade, and the widespread introduction of low cost, smokable cocaine, as freebase or crack, has had a devastating effect on all aspects of society, from school systems to drug treatment programs.[1] The psychiatric and medical sequelae of cocaine use are generally seen after 2-4 years of cocaine use.[2-4] The initial therapeutic management of the cocaine addict must deal with a wide range of physical and psychological withdrawal symptoms including depression, fatigue, anorexia, irritability, disturbed sleep, and a sometimes overwhelming craving for cocaine.[5,6] Until relatively recently, these symptoms were considered to be part of a psychological dependence on the drug, with recommended treatments characterized by a psychotherapeutic orientation.[7] Recent neurophysiologic evidence suggests, however, that these withdrawal symptoms may be the result of "neuroadaptation"[8] or direct physiological consequences of cocaine. Consequently, attention has begun to focus on the utility of pharmacologic agents as adjuncts to traditional treatment regimens.[9-11]

THE DOPAMINE DEPLETION HYPOTHESIS

Several different neurochemical phenomena have been posited as the substrate for post-cocaine withdrawal. One suggested physiological basis for cocaine withdrawal involves the depletion of dopamine.[9,12,13] It has been suggested that cocaine reward and euphoria result from the acute activation of the dopamine systems in the brain. While acute cocaine administration can produce a temporary increase in dopamine, chronic cocaine use results in neurotransmitter and neuroendocrine alterations. Dopamine depletion is hypothesized to result from overstimulation of these neurons and excessive synaptic metabolism of this neurotransmitter. Repeated cocaine administration produces an absolute decrease in brain dopamine that can be temporarily corrected by acute cocaine administration — "refreshing" the system only briefly while causing further depletion.[12]

Several pharmacotherapies have been developed on the basis of the dopamine depletion hypothesis. Bromocriptine (Parlodel) is a direct dopamine agonist that appears to facilitate binding of dopamine to postsynaptic receptors.[12] Bromocriptine appears to have no abuse potential in humans but is self-administered by animals.[10] Open clinical trials have provided preliminary evidence of the efficacy of bromocriptine in alleviating withdrawal symptoms and cocaine use,[14,15] and at least one study[16] has shown benefits of bromocriptine with methadone patients. A number of double-blind placebo controlled studies have shown bromocriptine to be effective in alleviating early cocaine withdrawal symptoms[17-22] and craving.[6,17] One advantage of bromocriptine (and amantadine, as reviewed below) is that the onset of action appears to be immediate.[11,17] A disadvantage of bromocriptine appears to be the "substantial spectrum" of side effects,[10,22] including nausea, headache and psychotogenic effects.

Bromcriptine has come to be recognized as a standard treatment of acute early withdrawal symptoms,[11,23] and may be of benefit in combination with tricyclic antidepressants.[19] Several studies, however, cast some doubt on the validity of the dopamine depletion hypothesis. In an uncontrolled trial of 25 heavy cocaine users,[24] measurements of pre- and post-bromocriptine serum prolactin levels, an indicator of inhibitory dopaminergic control, did not suggest dopamine depletion. Furthermore, the therapeutic effects of bromocriptine could not be differentiated from those of placebo. Two additional studies have assessed dopamine concentrations following long term cocaine administration in animals: one study[25] found *increased* dopamine concentration, the other[26] reported effects attributable only to the last cocaine dose.

Amantadine (Symmetrel) is a dopamimetic (i.e., dopamine mimicking) agent that increases dopaminergic transmission, although it is unclear whether its mechanism of action is in increasing dopamine release or decreasing uptake. Amantadine has been found effective in the treatment of early withdrawal symptoms in open clinical trials.[27-29] Double-blind studies have generally supported the effectiveness of amantadine,[20,22] although at least one double-blind study has reported negative results.[30] Amantadine is typically associated with fewer side effects than bromocriptine,[22] but reports of side effects may be dose-related. The onset of action for amantadine is unclear, with several studies reporting almost immediate onset of effect,[22,29] and at least one study reporting a 1-2 week lag.[28]

Methylphenidate (Ritalin), another dopamimetic agent, has also been suggested in the treatment of early withdrawal. Because methylphenidate has somewhat less abuse liability than cocaine, has a rapid onset of effect, and a longer duration of action, its use might parallel methadone treatment for heroin.[10] Early clinical trials supported the efficacy of methylphenidate.[31,32] However, later reports[33,34] cautioned against its use, citing tolerance, diminished anti-craving effects over time, and a sense of mild stimulation that evoked an increase in craving. An important exception to this caution is the use of methylphenidate for treatment of cocaine abuse among patients with Attention Deficit Disorder (ADD) residual type, where no secondary increase in craving, tolerance and rebound cocaine use has been reported.[31,32]

RECEPTOR SUPERSENSITIVITY

Gawin and Kleber[35] have hypothesized that chronic use of cocaine induces decreases in dopaminergic activity, mediated by supersensitivity of inhibitory dopaminergic auto-receptors. It is this phenomena that is suggested to be the neurochemical basis of post-cocaine dysphoria and craving, and consequently may be a major factor in failed attempts to end cocaine use. Auto-receptor super-sensitivity has been demonstrated experimentally in animals exposed to cocaine.[36]

Tricyclic antidepressants have been shown to reduce dopaminergic receptor sensitivity in animals,[37] this inducing beta-adrenergic subsensitivity.[38] It has therefore been hypothesized that tricyclic antidepressants may be effective in treating chronic cocaine withdrawal by reversing this cocaine-induced dopaminergic supersensitivity.[35,39]

Open clinical trials provided preliminary evidence that desipramine (Norpramin, Pertofrane) was effective in reducing craving and facilitating abstinence among "pure" cocaine users,[35,40] and among cocaine-abusing methadone patients.[41] Double-blind comparisons of desipramine with matched control groups[42] and with inactive[43] and active placebos[19,43,44] have supported the effectiveness of desipramine in the treatment of chronic cocaine withdrawal symptoms. One study has shown that adding desipramine to a bromocriptine regimen—a drug with a rapid onset of action—may enhance therapeutic effects.[19] Desipramine has generally shown a low incidence of side effects, low toxicity, high patient acceptance and absence of abuse potential.[10,17]

There is preliminary evidence that other antidepressants, most notably imipramine,[45,46] trazadone[47,48] and maprotiline[49] may also be of some benefit in the treatment of chronic withdrawal.

The principal disadvantage to tricyclic antidepressants appears to be the delayed onset of action, ranging from 10 days to several weeks.[10,11,17,35] Fishman and Foltin[50] noted that desipramine maintenance at 3-4 weeks had no effect on human cocaine self-administration, while being associated with significant increases in blood pressure and heart rate. At least two short term double-blind studies of low dose desipramine have failed to demonstrate therapeutic efficacy in comparison to placebo.[51,52]

BENZODIAZEPINES AND NEUROLEPTICS

One area in which pharmacological therapy is indicated is in the treatment of acute sequelae of cocaine use: severe symptoms of cocaine intoxication such as agitation, anxiety and paranoia, and psychotic disorders which can occur with cocaine abuse. Long-acting benzodiazepines (e.g., diazepam, chlordiazepoxide, oxazepam, clonazepam) have been recommended for the treatment of severe "crash" symptoms of cocaine intoxication and withdrawal[53] and are frequently useful in controlling symptoms for several days after a heavy cocaine binge.[11] One caveat in the use of benzodiazepines is their ready potential for abuse, especially in a demonstrated abuse-prone population. Short-acting benzodiazepines particularly have shown considerable abuse potential and are not recommended for use in this population.[53] Other benzodiazepines, particularly oxazepam, have shown far less abuse potential and may be an effective component in the early treatment of crash symptoms.[54,55]

Neuroleptics have been recommended in the treatment of severe cocaine withdrawal when psychotic symptoms are present.[53] However, certain safeguards must be taken in the use of neuroleptics. It has been suggested that neuroleptics may increase or intensify hyperthermia associated with cocaine overdoses.[56-58] Also, studies with animals have shown that different neuroleptics (e.g., haloperidol and fluphenazine) may differentially effect mesolimbic dopamine receptors,[59] potentially leading to differences in efficacy of treating these cocaine crash symptoms.[11] Further, neuroleptics also may produce anhedonia, thereby making compliance problematic.[10]

One agent with neuroleptic activity has received recent attention. Flupenthixol is a depot xanthene derivative not currently available for research or clinical applications in the U.S., which has been used for over a decade in Europe, the Far East, and the Caribbean. At low doses it appears to have rapid antidepressant activity and has not been associated with tardive dyskinesia;[60-62] at higher doses it has neuroleptic activity, blocking dopamine binding with substantial activity at D-1, D-2, and inhibitory D-2 auto receptors.[63]

Neuroleptics and other dopamine blocking agents diminish stimulant effects in animals, presumably by blocking post synaptic receptor dopamine binding.[64] However, low dose neuroleptics (e.g., phenothiazines, butyrophenones) appear to exacerbate stimulant withdrawal symptoms and fail to block stimulant effects.[64-66] Gawin and Ellinwood[67] have hypothesized that cocaine induces a decrease in dopaminergic activity, mediated by supersensitivity of inhibitory dopaminergic auto receptors that contribute to the stimulant withdrawal syndrome. They speculate that flupenthixol in low doses may demonstrate greater affinity for dopamine auto receptors than post-synaptic receptors, preferentially binding to these inhibitory sites. The resultant increase in dopaminergic activity would account for its antidepressant effects. At higher doses and plasma concentrations, as effects on post-synaptic receptors prevail, neuroleptic-like activity may result in cocaine blocking.

A preliminary report[68] provides evidence of the successful use of flupenthixol decanoate in the treatment of 10 crack smoking outpatients at the Princess Margaret Hospital in Nassau, Bahamas. Nine of 10 subjects reported reduction of cocaine craving within three days of flupenthixol administration, and all nine had eliminated crack use by the second week. Treatment retention for these patients was significantly improved as well. Double-blind trials of flupenthixol are now underway.

COCAINE-INDUCED KINDLING

An alternative physiological basis for cocaine craving may be that of kindling—the progressive facilitation of neuronal activity in discrete regions of the brain elicited by temporally spaced exposure to specific pharmacologic or electrical stimuli.[69,70] Several researchers[70-73] have demonstrated that the administration of psychostimulants, including cocaine, is associated with multi-stage kindling effects (e.g., stereotypic behaviors, disruption in learning) eventually leading to a major seizure activity. It has been hypothesized that kindling is the physiological mechanism responsible for the subjective experience of craving associated with cocaine use.[74] Because of its mechanism of action as an anticonvulsant, carbamazepine has been suggested as an agent beneficial in reversing kindling, thereby eliminating craving.[75]

Carbamazepine is a chemical compound that has proven highly effective in the treatment of a variety of seizure disorders,[76,77] and more recently, affective disorders[78,79] and temporal lobe syndromes.[80] In generalized seizures thought to arise from the limbic system and the temperal lobe, and in complex partial seizures, carbamazepine has been an especially effective treatment.[77,81] In animals, carbamazepine has been show to selectively inhibit early, developmental phases of pharmacological kindling induced by local anesthetics,[82] and block late phases of electrically kindled seizures in animals.[82]

A separate line of research has demonstrated that carbamazepine has similar but largely opposite effects to those of cocaine on neurotransmitter systems. Carbamazepine has been shown to increase dopamine concentration in brain slices[83] and cerebroventricular perfusates,[84] block synaptosomal norepinephrine reuptake,[85] increase the firing rate of locus cereleus neurons,[86] increase plasma tryptophan,[87] and increase acetylcholine levels in the striatum.[88]

Recent studies conducted at the University of Minnesota suggest that carbamazepine may be useful in alleviating craving for cocaine, and therefore may be of benefit as an adjunct to traditional treatment regimens. An open clinical trial involving 35 outpatients showed a significant reduction in cocaine use (62.1 days per 100 use prior to treatment compared to 18.3 days per 100 use while in treatment; t = 3.5; p < .001) among the 17 highly compliant patients. A preliminary report on these findings has been published.[75]

An intensive case study of two VA Medical Center cocaine-using methadone maintenance patients[89] provides further evidence of the efficacy of carbamazepine. Urinalysis results indicated that both patients were able to abstain from cocaine while on carbamazepine: one patient for the final 6 months of the trial and the other for the final 3 1/2 months of the trials.

The first systematically controlled study of carbamazepine in the treatment of cocaine abuse was recently completed at the University of Minnesota.[90] The study was a 20-day, randomized, double-blind, placebo-controlled "cross-over" study involving 32 unmotivated, paid crack users. Subjects reported for 22 consecutive days including screen and baseline visits. Each day subjects provided a daily urine sample and completed self-report ratings forms. Blood samples were taken at screen, and days 5, 10, 15 and 20. Blind medication was dispensed daily, and subjects were required to take the medication in the presence of the clinical staff. Subjects received 10 consecutive days of placebo and 10 consecutive days of carbamazepine, with the order of drug randomized. One-half of the subjects received a daily dose of 200 mg; the other half received 400 mg. The analysis of the daily urine samples provided clear support for the short-term effectiveness of carbamazepine. The average number of positive urines based on nine days of observation (the first and last day on carbamazepine were eliminated from statistical analysis to eliminate potential "carry-over" effects) was 6.8 for carbamazepine days compared to 7.5 for placebo days (F = 4.44; df = 31,1; p = .043). Longer term double-blind placebo-controlled studies are now in progress at several sites.

THE TREATMENT OF COCAINE-ABUSING
METHADONE PATIENTS

One particularly distressing aspect of the recent cocaine epidemic has been the relapse of stable former heroin users now in successful methadone maintenance programs around the nation.[91] Several reports indicate that cocaine abuse among this population may be as high as 70%.[92,93] While methadone diminishes or eliminates the pleasurable effects of heroin, thereby extinguishing its reinforcing properties, methadone may have quite the opposite effect on the pleasurable aspects of cocaine. When using cocaine by itself, opiate users often report a somewhat dysphoric experience. In contrast, when mixing cocaine with an opioid agonist such as methadone or heroin, a so-called "speedball," the experience is reported by being quite pleasant and reinforcing.[93]

Several adjunctive pharmacologic agents have been suggested in the treatment of cocaine abusing methadone patients. Two open clinical trials have suggested that carbamazepine may be effective in the treatment of cocaine abuse among methadone maintenance patients.[75,89] They found, however, that carbamazepine stimulated the metabolism of methadone, thereby inducing a relative withdrawal state in some patients before the next methadone dose. Clinically, drugs which inhibit this enzyme, such as cimetidine, appear to eliminate this relative withdrawal state at hours 18-24. Alternatively, Halikas et al. have suggested slow induction of carbamazepine with a corresponding increase in methadone dose of 5-15 milligrams.[94] Preliminary studies have also indicated that despramine[41,95] and amantadine[27] may be of use in treating cocaine abuse among methadone patients.

All of the drugs described presumably work by decreasing cocaine craving or by blocking the acute effects of cocaine administration. An alternative pharmacologic approach for this population may be to seek different opioid maintenance agents which do not produce this "speed ball" effect. Two alternative maintenance agents have been suggested.[96,97] Buprenorphine is a partial opioid antagonist whose relatively lower agonist actions may decrease the speedball interaction with cocaine. Buprenorphine has been shown to be effective in the detoxification from opioid dependence.[98,99] Since buprenorphine's antagonist activity appears to increase at higher doses, it has been speculated that cocaine abuse might be lower at higher buprenorphine doses.[99] The other opioid antagonist that has received some attention is naltrexone. Naltrexone is a long-acting competitive opioid antagonist that blocks the positive reinforcement of administered opioids by preventing them from binding to the opioid receptor.[100,101] Two recent reports by Kosten and colleagues[96,97] provide preliminary evidence that cocaine use among patients maintained on buprenorphine or naltrexone may be significantly lower than comparable patients maintained on methadone.

SEROTONIN ANTAGONISTS

Still another possible mechanism of cocaine reinforcement may be related to the neurotransmitter, serotonin. Acute cocaine use has been found to inhibit serotonin activity,[102] and it has been suggested that these serotonin alterations may be responsible for the acute insomnia seen in cocaine intoxication and hypersomnia associated with cocaine withdrawal.[9] Serotonergic agents (e.g., Sertratine, Fluvoxamine, Fluoxetine, trazadone, L-tryptophan) may prove to be of benefit in the treatment of cocaine addicts by increasing serotonin. However, the data with respect to the effectiveness of serotonergic agents is largely anecdotal to this point.[46,48] Open-label and double-blind studies are currently in progress.

FUTURE DIRECTIONS
IN PHARMACOTHERAPEUTIC INTERVENTIONS

Cocaine abuse in clinical populations, controlled laboratory settings, and animal models, is being more intensely and thoroughly studied than any previous drug abuse epidemic. New clues and connections are daily suggested which may lead to more effective treatment regimens. Clinical studies will need to document the differential patterns of cocaine use seen, and the different diagnostic populations using cocaine, so that, as new treatments are developed, their precise usefulness can be clearly demonstrated.

As animal studies progress, cocaine effects will be more narrowly and clearly defined. The immediate neuropharmacologic effects of cocaine may have an impact on reinforcement and establishment of use, while repeated use may have long-term neurophysiological consequences which perpetuate drug seeking behavior or other personality changes. In short, future studies may serve to further document the clinically apparent observation that the immediate effects of cocaine are different from the long-term consequences of use.

As an array of useful medications is defined, and precise populations and patterns of use are identified, specific indications of use for each medication will be clarified. Clinical consensus is already developing regarding the practicality of various medications in different settings: inpatient versus outpatient, short-term versus long-term, etc. It is likely that, in the intermediate term, a "cascade" of medications will be identified for varying types of cocaine users, such that some medications will be used alone, some will be used sequentially, and some will be used in tandem.

Another important insight developing in this treatment research arena, is an acknowledgment of the limited usefulness of pharmacotherapy in the treatment of a condition which begins in human behavior. While presumably driven by as yet not understood biological forces, the behavior of drug use is, at first, voluntary, the impact on the individual and their world is wide spread and far reaching, and the consequences are so overwhelming as to require a psychological and psychosocial framework for the recovery process. Thus, to be maximally accepted and effective, pharmacotherapy must be used within the context of the current standard of psychosocial, rehabilitative care, and the current reliance on abstinence-oriented peer group counseling.

REFERENCES

1. National Institute on Drug Abuse: *Proceedings of Community Epidemiology Work Group.* NIDA Division of Epidemiology and Prevention, June, 1989.

2. Adams, E.H. & Kozel, N.J. Cocaine use in America: Introduction and overview. In E.H. Adams & N.J. Kozel (Eds.), *Cocaine Use in America: Epidemiologic and Clinical Perspectives.* National Institute of Drug Abuse Research Monograph Series, 1985, 61:35-49.

3. Kleber, H.D. & Gawin, F. The spectrum of cocaine use and its treatment. *Journal of Clinical Psychiatry*, 1984, 45(12):18-23.

4. Schnoll, S.H., Karrigan, J., Kitchen, S.B., Daghestani, A. & Hansen, T. Characteristics of cocaine abusers presenting for treatment. In E.H. Adams & N.J. Kozel (Eds.), *Cocaine Use in America: Epidemiologic and Clinical Perspectives.* NIDA Research Monograph Series, 1985, 61: 171-181.

5. Dackis, C.A., Gold, M.S. & Sweeney, D.R. The physiology of cocaine craving and "crashing." *Archives of General Psychiatry*, 1987, 44:298-299.

6. Dackis, C.A., Gold, M.S., Sweeney, D.R., Byron, J.P. & Climko, R. Single-dose bromocriptine reverses cocaine craving. *Psychiatry Research*, 1987, 20: 261-264.

7. Grinspoon, L. & Bakalar, J.B. Drug dependence: Non-narcotic agents.

In H.I. Kaplan, A.M. Freedman & B.J. Sadock (Eds.), *Comprehensive Textbook of Psychiatry, 3rd Edition*, Baltimore: Williams & Wilkins, 1980.

8. Gawin, F.H. & Kleber, H.D. Abstinence symptomatology and psychiatric diagnosis in cocaine abusers: Clinical observations. *Archives of General Psychiatry*, 1986, 41: 107-113.

9. Dackis, C.A. & Gold, M.S. Psychopharmacology of cocaine. *Psychiatric Annals*, 1988, 18(9):528-530.

10. Gawin, F.H. Chronic neuropharmacology of cocaine: Progress in pharmacotherapy. *Journal of Clinical Psychiatry*, 1988, 49 (2 suppl.), 11-16.

11. Kosten, T.R. Pharmacotherapeutic interventions for cocaine abuse. *Journal of Nervous and Mental Disease*, 1989 (7), 177:379-389.

12. Dackis, C.A. & Gold, M.S. New concepts in cocaine addiction: The dopamine depletion hypothesis. *Neuroscience and Biobehavioral Reviews*, 1985, 9: 469-477.

13. Wyatt, R.J., Karoum, F., Suddath, R. & Hitri, A. The role of dopamine in cocaine use and abuse. *Psychiatric Annals*, 1988, 18(9), 528-530.

14. Dackis, C.A. & Gold, M.S. Bromocriptine as a treatment for cocaine abuse. *Lancet*, 1985, 1: 1151-1152.

15. Extein, I.L., Gross, D.A. & Gold, M.S. Bromocriptine treatment of cocaine withdrawal symptoms (letter). *American Journal of Psychiatry*, 1989, 146(3):403.

16. Kosten, R.T. Schumann, B. & Wright, D. Bromocriptine treatment of cocaine abuse in methadone maintained patients (letter). *American Journal of Psychiatry*, 1988, 145: 381-382.

17. Extein, I.L. & Gold, M.S. The treatment of cocaine addicts: Bromocriptine or desipramine? *Psychiatric Annals*, 1988, 18(9):535-537.

18. Giannini, A.J., Baumgartel, P. & DiMarzio, L.R. Bromocriptine therapy in cocaine withdrawal. *Journal of Clinical Pharmacology*, 1987, 27(4):267-270.

19. Giannini, A.J. & Billet, W. Bromocriptine-desipramine protocol in the treatment of cocaine addiction. *Journal of Clinical Pharmacology*, 1987, 27(8):549-554.

20. Giannini, A.J., Folts, D.J., Feather, J.N. & Sullivan, B.S. Bromocriptine and amantadine in cocaine detoxification. *Psychiatry Research*, 1989, 29(1):11-16.

21. Kumor, K., Sherer, M. & Jaffe, J. Effects of bromocriptine pretreatment on subjective and physiological responses to intravenous cocaine. *Pharmacology, Biochemistry and Behavior*, 1989, 33(4):829-837.

22. Tennant, F.S. & Sagherian, A.A. Double-blind comparison of amantadine and bromocriptine for ambulatory withdrawal from cocaine dependence. *Archives of Internal Medicine*, 1987, 147(1):109-112.

23. Sitland-Marken, P.A., Wells, B.G., Froemming, J.H., Chu, C.C. & Brown, C.S. Psychiatric applications of bromocriptine therapy. *Journal of Clinical Psychiatry*, 1990, 51(2):68-82.

24. Teller, D.W. & Devenyi, P. Bromocriptine in cocaine withdrawal: Does it work? *International Journal of Addictions*, 1988, 23(11):1197-1205.

25. Roy, S.N., Bhattacharyya, A.K., Pradhan, S. & Pradhan, S.N. Behavioral and neurochemical effects of repeated administration of cocaine in rats. *Neuropharmacology*, 1978, 17:559-564.

26. Ho, B.T., Taylor, D.L. & Estevez, V.S. Behavioral effects of cocaine: Metabolic and neurochemical approach. In E.H. Ellinwood & M.M. Kilby (Eds.), *Cocaine and Other Stimulants*. New York: Plenum Publishing Corp., 1977.

27. Handelmann, L., Chordia, P.L., Escovar, I.L., Marion, I.J. & Lowenson, J. Amantadine for treatment of cocaine dependence in methadone-maintained patients (letter). *American Journal of Psychiatry*, 1988, 145(4):533.

28. Handelmann, L., Lowenson, J., Marion, I. et al. Amantadine treatment of cocaine abuse. *National Institute of Drug Abuse Research Monograph Series*. 1988.

29. Morgan, C., Kosten, T., Gawin, F. & Kleber, H. Pilot trial of amantadine for ambulatory withdrawal from cocaine dependence. *National Institute of Drug Abuse Research Monograph Series*, 1988, 81:81-85.

30. Gawin, F.H., Morgan, C., Kosten, T.R. & Kleber, H.D. Double-blind evaluation of the effect of acute amantadine on cocaine craving. *Psychopharmacology*, 1989, 97(3):402-403.

31. Khatzian, E.J. Cocaine dependence: An extreme case and marked improvement with methylphenidate treatment. *American Journal of Psychiatry*, 1983, 140:784-785.

32. Khatzian, E.J., Gawin, F.H., Kleber, H.D. & Riordan, C. Methylphenidate treatment of cocaine dependence: A preliminary report. *Journal of Substance Abuse Treatment*, 1984, 107-112.

33. Crowley, T.J. Cautionary note on methylphenidate for cocaine dependence (letter). *American Journal of Psychiatry*, 1984, 141(2):327-328.

34. Gawin, F.H., Riordan, C. & Kleber, H.D. Methylphenidate use in non-ADD cocaine users: A negative study. *American Journal of Drug and Alcohol Abuse*, 1985, 11:193-197.

35. Gawin, F.H. & Kleber, H.D. Cocaine abuse treatment: Open pilot trial with desipramine and lithium carbonate. *Archives of General Psychiatry*, 1984, 41:903-909.

36. Dwoskin, L.P., Peris, J., Yasuda, R.P., Philpott, K. & Zahniser, N.R. Repeated cocaine administration results in supersensitivity of striatal D-2 dopamine receptors to pergolide. *Life Science*, 1988, 42:255-262.

37. Koide, T. & Matshushita, H. An enhanced sensitivity of muscarinic cholinergic receptor associated with dopaminergic receptor subsensitivity after chronic antidepressant treatment. *Life Science*, 1981, 28:1139-1145.

38. Banerjee, S.P., King, L.S., Riggi, S.J. & Chanda, S.K. Development of beta-adrenergic receptor subsensitivity by anti-depressants. *Nature*, 1977, 268:455-456.

39. Dewitt, H. & Wise, R.A. A blockade of cocaine reinforcement in rats

with the dopamine blocker pimozide but not with the noradrenergic blockers phenolamine or phenoxybenzamine. *Canadian Journal of Psychology*, 1977, 31:195-203.

40. Tennant, F.S. & Rawson, R.A. Cocaine and amphetamine dependence treated with desipramine. *National Institute of Drug Abuse Research Monograph Series*, 1983, 43:351-355.

41. Kosten, R.T., Schumann, B., Wright, D., Carney, M.K. & Gawin, F.H. A preliminary study of desipramine in the treatment of cocaine abuse in methadone maintenance patients. *Journal of Clinical Psychiatry*, 1987, 48: 442-444.

42. O'Brien, C.P., Childress, A.R., Arndt, I.A., McLellan, A.T., Woody, G.E. & Maany, I. Pharmacological and behavioral treatments of cocaine dependence: Controlled studies. *Journal of Clinical Psychiatry*, 1988, 49(2 suppl.), 17-22.

43. Gawin, F.H., Kleber, H.D., Byck, R., Rounsaville, B.J., Kosten, T.R., Jatlow, P.I. & Morgan, C. Desipramine facilitation of initial cocaine abstinence. *Archives of General Psychiatry*, 1989, 46:117-121.

44.. Giannini, A.J., Malone, D.A., Giannini, M.C., Price, W.A. & Loiselle, R.H. Treatment of depression in chronic cocaine and phencyclidine abuse with desipramine. *Journal of Clinical Pharmacology*, 1986, 26:211-214.

45. Huyghe, P. A cure for cocaine? *New York Magazine*, 1984, 74-84.

46. Rosecan, J. *The treatment of cocaine abuse with imipramine, L-tyrosine, and L-tryptophan*. Presented at World Congress of Psychiatry, Vienna, July 14-19, 1983.

47. Rowbotham, M., Jones, R.T., Benowitz, N. & Jacob, P. Trazodone-oral cocaine interactions. *Archives of General Psychiatry*, 1984, 41:895-899.

48. Small, G.W. & Purcell, J.J. Trazodone and cocaine abuse. *Archives of General Psychiatry*, 1985, 42:524.

49. Brotman, A.W., Witkie, S.M., Gelenberg, A.J., Falk, W.E., Wojcik, J. & Leahy, L. An open trial of maprotiline for the treatment of cocaine abuse: A pilot study. *Journal of Clinical Pharmacology*, 1988, 8(2):125-127.

50. Fishman, M.W. & Foltin, R.W. Interaction of desipramine maintenance with cocaine self-administration in humans. *Abstracts of the 27th Annual Meeting of American College of Neuropsychopharmacology*, 1988, December 11-16, San Juan, Puerto Rico.

51. Tennant, F.S. Double-blind comparison of desipramine and placebo in withdrawal from cocaine dependence. *National Institute of Drug Abuse Research Monograph Series*, 1984, 55: 159-163.

52. Tennant, F.S. & Tarver, A.L. Double-blind comparison of desipramine and placebo in withdrawal from cocaine dependence. *National Institute of Drug Abuse Research Monograph Series*, 1984, 55: 159-163.

53. Millman, R.B. Evaluation and clinical management of cocaine abusers. *Journal of Clinical Pharmacology*, 1988, 49(2 suppl.): 1988.

54. Owen, R.T. & Tyrer, P. Benzodiazepine dependence: A review of the evidence. *Drugs*, 1983, 25: 385-398.

55. Woody, G.E., O'Brien, C.P. & Greenstein, R. Misuse and abuse of diazepam: An increasingly common medical problem. *International Journal of Addiction*, 1975, 10:843-848.

56. Kosten, T.R. & Kleber, H.D. Sudden death in cocaine abusers: Relation to neuroleptic malignant syndrome? *Lancet*, 1987, 1:1198-1199.

57. Kosten, T.R. & Kleber, H.D. Rapid death during cocaine abuse: Variant of neuroleptic malignant syndrome? *American Journal of Alcohol Abuse*, 1988, 12:1-16.

58. Mittleman, R. & Wetli, C.V. Death caused by recreational cocaine use. *Journal of the American Medical Association*, 1984, 252: 1889-1892.

59. Thierry, A.M., LeDouarin, C. & Penit, J. Variation in the ability of neuroleptics to block the inhibitory influence of dopaminergic neurons in the activity of cells in the rat prefrontal cortex. *Brain Research Bulletin*, 1986, 16: 155-160.

60. Baldwin, R., Cranfield, R. & Swarbrick, D.J. A double-blind trial comparing single and divided daily doses of flupenthixol in the treatment of mild to moderately severe depression: A multicentre trial in general practice. *Journal of Int. Biomet. Inform. Data*, 1983, 4: 37-42.

61. Frolund, F. Treatment of depression in general practice: A controlled trial of flupenthixol. *Current Medical Research Opin.*, 1974, 2:78-89.

62. Poldinger, W. & Sieberns, S. Depression-inducing and antidepressive effects of neuroleptics: Experiences with flupenthixol and flupenthixol decanoate. *Neuropsychobiology*, 1983, 10:131-136.

63. Robertson, M.M. & Trimble, M.R. Major tranquilizers used as antidepressants. *Journal of Affective Disorders*, 1982, 4: 173-195.

64. Wise, R. Neural mechanisms of the reinforcing action of cocaine. *NIDA Research Monograph Series, Volume 50*, 1984, U.S. Government Printing Office; Washington, D.C., pp. 15-53.

65. Gawin, F.H. Neuroleptic reduction of cocaine-induced paranoia but not euphoria? *Psychopharmacology*, 1986, 90: 142-143.

66. Scherer, M., Kumor, K. & Jaffe, J. Effects of intravenous cocaine are partially attenuated by haloperidol. *Psych. Research*, 1989.

67. Gawin, F.H. & Ellinwood, E.H. Cocaine and other stimulants — actions, abuse and treatment. *New England Journal of Medicine*, 1988, 318: 1173-1182.

68. Gawin, F.H., Allen, D. & Humblestone, B. Outpatient treatment of 'crack' cocaine smoking with flupenthixol decanoate: A preliminary report. *Archives of General Psychiatry*, 1989, 46(4):322-325.

69. Goddard, G.V., McIntyre, D.C. & Leach, C.K. A permanent change in brain functioning resulting from daily electrical stimulation. *Experimental Neurology*, 1969, 25: 295.

70. Post, R.M. & Kopanda, R.T. Cocaine, kindling & psychosis. *American Journal of Psychiatry*, 1976, 133: 627-634.

71. Eidelberg, E., Lesse, H. & Gault, F.P. An experimental model of temperal lobe epilepsy: Studies of the convulsant properties of cocaine. In G.H. Glaser (ed.). *EEG and Behavior*, New York: Basic Books, 1963.

72. Ellinwood, E.H. & Kilbey, M.M. Chronic stimulant intoxication models of psychosis. In E. Hanlin & E. Usdin, *Animal Models in Psychiatry and Neurology*, New York: Pergamon Press, 1977.

73. Post, R.M., Kopanda, R.T. & Black, K.E. Progressive effects of cocaine on behavior and central amine metabolism in rhesus monkeys: Relationship to kindling and psychosis. *Biological Psychiatry*, 1976, 11: 403-419.

74. Halikas, J.A. & Kuhn, K.L. A possible neurophysiologial basis of cocaine craving. *Annals of Clinical Psychiatry*, 1990, 2(2): 79-83.

75. Halikas, J.A., Kemp, K.D., Kuhn, K.L., Carlson, G.A. & Crea, F.S. Carbamazepine for cocaine addiction? Letter to the editor. *Lancet*, 1989, March 18, 623-624.

76. Penry, J.K. & Daly, D.D. Complex and partial seizures and their treatment. In *Advances in Neurology, Volume 11*, 1975, New York: Raven Press.

77. Porter, R.J. & Penry, J.K. Efficacy in choice of anti-epileptic drugs. In H. Meinardi & A.J. Rowan (Eds.), *Advances in Epileptology: Psychology, Pharmacotherapy and New Diagnostic Approaches*, 1978, Amsterdam: Swets and Zeitlinger.

78. Ballenger, J.C. & Post, R.M. Therapeutic effects of carbamazepine in affective illness: A preliminary report. *Clinical Psychopharmacology*, 1978, 2: 159-175.

79. Post, R.M., Uhde, T.W. & Roy-Byrne, P.P. Correlates of antimanic responses to carbamazepine, 1987, *Psychiatry Research*, 1987, 21: 71-83.

80. Porter, R.J. & Theodore, W.H. Nonsedative regimens in the treatment of epilepsy. *Archives of Internal Medicine*, 1983, 143:945-947.

81. Callaghan, N., Kenny, R.A. & O'Neill, B. A prospective study between carbamazepine, phenytoin, and sodium valproate as monotherapy in previously untreated and recently diagnosed patients with epilepsy. *Journal of Neurol Neurosurg Psychiatry*, 1985, 48: 639-644.

82. Post, R.M. Time course of clinical effects of carbamazepine: Implication for mechanism of action. *Journal of Clinical Psychiatry*, 1988, 49 (suppl): 4, 35-46.

83. Keneko, S., Kurahashi, K., Mori, A., Hill, R.G. & Taberner, P.V. The mechanisms of actions of carbamazepine. In *International Congress Series (Abstracts of the 12th World Congress of Neurology*, 1981, Princeton: Excerpta Medica, 548: 318-319.

84. Kawalik, S., Levitt, M. & Barkai, A. Effects of carbamazepine and antidepressant drugs on endogenous catecholamine levels in the cerebroventricular compartment of the rat. *Psychopharmacology*, 1984, 83: 169-171.

85. Purdy, R.E., Julien, R.M., Rairhust, A.S. & Terry, M.D. Effect of carbamazepine on the vitro uptake and release of norepinephrine in adrenergic nerves of rabbit aorta and in whole brain synaptosomes. *Epilepsia*, 1977, 18: 251-257.

86. Olpe, H.R. & Jones, R.S. The action of anticonvulsant drugs on the firing of locus cereleus neurons: Selective, activating effect of carbamazepine. *European Journal of Pharmacology*, 1983, 91:107-110.

87. Pratt, J.A., Jenner, P., Johnson, A.L., Shorvon, S.D. & Reynolds, E.H. Anticonvulsant drugs alter plasma tryptophan concentrations in epileptic patients: Implications for antiepileptic action and mental function. *Journal of Neurol Neurosurg Psychiatry*, 1984, 47:1131.

88. Consolo, S., Bianchi, S. & Ladinsky, H. Effect of carbamazepine on cholinergic parameters in rat brain areas. *Neuropharmacology*, 1976, 15:653-657.

89. Halikas, J.A., Kuhn, K.L. & Maddux, T.L. Reduction of cocaine use among methadone maintenance patients using concurrent carbamazepine maintenance. *Annals of Clinical Psychiatry*, 1990, 2(1), 3-6.

90. Halikas, J.A., Crosby, R.D., Carlson, G.A., Crea, F.S., Graves, N.M. & Bowers, L.D. Cocaine reduction in unmotivated crack users using carbamazepine versus placebo in a short-term, double-blind crossover design. *Clinical Pharmacology and Therapeutics, 1991*, 50, in press.

91. Cushman, P. Effects of a cocaine epidemic on a population of methadone maintenance maintained drug abusers. *Substance Abuse*, 1988, 9(1):46-50.

92. Kosten, T.R., Gawin, F.H., Rounsaville, B.J., Kleber, H.D. Cocaine abuse among opioid addicts: Demographic and diagnostic factors in treatment. *American Journal of Drug and Alcohol abuse*, 1986, 12: 1-16, 1986.

93. Kosten, T.R, Rounsaville, B.J. & Kleber, H.D. A 2.5 year follow-up of cocaine use among treated opioid addicts: Have our treatments helped? *Archives of General Psychiatry*, 1987, 44: 281-284.

94. Kuhn, K.L., Halikas, J.A. & Kemp, K.D. Carbamazepine treatment of cocaine dependence in methadone maintenance patients with dual opiate-cocaine addiction. *NIDA Research Monograph Series: Problems of Drug Dependence*, 1989, 95: 316-317.

95. Kosten, R.T., Gawin, F. & Schumann, B. Treating cocaine abusing methadone maintenance patients with desipramine. *NIDA Research Monograph Series*, 1988, 81: 237-241.

96. Kosten, T.R., Kleber, H.D. & Morgan, C.H. Treatment of cocaine abuse with buprenorphine. *Biological Psychiatry*, 1989a, 26: 637-639.

97. Kosten, T.R., Kleber, H.D. & Morgan, C.H. Role of opioid antagonists in treating intravenous cocaine abuse. *Life Sciences*, 1989b, 44(13):887-892.

98. Kosten, T.R. Buprenorphine detoxification from opioid dependence: A pilot study. *Life Sciences*, 1988, 42: 635-641.

99. Lewis, J.W. Buprenorphine. *Drug and Alcohol Dependency*, 1985, 14: 363-372.

100. Herridge, P. & Gold, M.S. Pharmacological adjuncts in the treatment of

opioid and cocaine addicts. *Journal of Psychoactive Drugs*, 1988, 20(3): 233-242.

101. Gonzalez, J.P. & Brogden, R.N. Naltrexone: A review of its pharmacodynamic and pharmacokinetic properties and therapeutic efficacy in the management of opioid dependence. *Drugs*, 1988, 35(3): 192-213.

102. Taylor, D. & Ho, B.T. Neurochemical effects of cocaine following acute repeated injection. *Journal of Neurosci. Research*, 1977, 3: 95-101.

Changes in Cocaine Use After Entry to Methadone Treatment

Stephen Magura, PhD
Qudsia Siddiqi, PhD
Robert C. Freeman, MA
Douglas S. Lipton, PhD

SUMMARY. A cohort sample of 93 addicts admitted to methadone maintenance in four clinics was followed-up for one year to determine change, and predictors of change, in cocaine use. Any use of cocaine in the preceding month decreased from 84% of subjects at admission to 66% at follow-up, and mean days of cocaine use per month for those still using decreased from 16 days to 9 days. Any drug injection in the preceding month decreased from 100% of sub-

Stephen Magura is Deputy Director of Research, Qudsia Siddiqi was Assistant Project Director, Robert C. Freeman was Research Associate, and Douglas S. Lipton is Director of Research, Narcotic and Drug Research, Inc.

This study was supported by Grant No. 5 R01 DA03991 (Project MERCURY) from the National Institute on Drug Abuse. The opinions expressed herein do not necessarily reflect the positions or policies of the cooperating institutions.

The authors are grateful to the following methadone programs in New York City for their cooperation in this study: Lower East Side Service Center (Units 1 and 3), Van Etten Drug Treatment Program, Beth Israel Medical Center (St. Luke's clinic), and New York Hospital Methadone Maintenance Program. Special thanks are extended to Edward M. Brown (Executive Director), Herbert Barish (Associate Director) and Joseph Krasnansky (Clinic Director), of the Lower East Side; Dr. Edward Shollar (Director) and Ronald Salon (Associate Director) of Van Etten; Nina Peyser (Director of Substance Abuse Planning) and Robert Dash (Clinic Director) of Beth Israel; and Aaron Wells (Medical Director) and Elizabeth Payne (Clinic Administrator) of New York Hospital.

EMIT is a trademark of SYVA Company.

Reprint requests may be addressed to Stephen Magura, PhD, Narcotic and Drug Research, Inc., 11 Beach Street, New York, NY 10013.

jects at admission to 39% at follow-up, among those remaining in the program. Continuance/cessation of cocaine use was not associated with program retention, but cocaine users were more likely to be administratively discharged. Reported symptoms of depression and speedballing at admission were significant predictors of continuance/cessation of cocaine use at follow-up. State-of-the-art cocaine abuse treatment, with attention to treatment of depression, would enhance the value of methadone maintenance for patients with dual heroin/cocaine addiction.

INTRODUCTION

Methadone maintenance is the largest drug abuse treatment modality in the United States, with about 75,000 narcotic addicts enrolled at any one time. Previous evaluative research has documented the effectiveness of methadone treatment for reducing participants' intravenous drug use, reducing their criminal behavior, and increasing their social productivity.[1-6] Reduction of intravenous drug use is especially important in view of the continuing AIDS epidemic. Moreover, numerous studies have shown that enrollment in methadone treatment, as well as longer length of treatment, are associated with lower HIV seroprevalence rates.[7-12]

The greatest single problem challenging methadone treatment today is the substantial increase in secondary substance abuse among patients, especially cocaine injection and crack use. Three recent multi-clinic studies found that 36% of patients used cocaine in a prior week,[13] 45% used in a prior month[14] and 51% used in a prior 6-month period.[15] In 1985 49% of addicts admitted to 6 methadone programs in New York, Baltimore and Philadelphia reported cocaine use in the preceding month,[16] and in 1989 75% of the 6,150 addicts admitted to all methadone programs in New York City reported cocaine as their "secondary substance" of abuse.[17] A 1989 survey of 15 methadone clinics nationwide found that cocaine use characterized up to 40% of patients enrolled for more than 6 months in several of the clinics studied.[18] The marked increase in cocaine use during the 1980's is clearly revealed in a trend study of urinalysis profiles for a single large methadone program in New York City. In 1981 only 21% of patients had at least one cocaine-positive urine, while in 1988 63% were found to be positive; the percentage of all urines taken that were cocaine-positive also increased.[10] High levels of cocaine/crack abuse among patients are turning media and public opinion against methadone.[19-21]

Cocaine abuse among methadone patients carries serious AIDS risks. The intravenous route of administration (either alone or together with heroin) remains predominant among cocaine abusing patients, although crack use is also becoming substantial, as this paper will show. Intravenous use of cocaine places patients, their drug-using peers and their sexual partners at risk for HIV transmission through needle sharing and unprotected sexual relations. Nearly a decade into the AIDS epidemic, a current national survey of intravenous drug users indicates that 84% continue to share needles, that only 32% use new or effectively-cleaned needles/works, and that 87% engage in unprotected sex.[22] A recent multi-program study of methadone patients who continued to inject drugs (primarily cocaine) during treatment found that 40% were sharing needles/works and 50% were not cleaning injection equipment consistently or effectively.[23] Cocaine injection is one of the strongest predictors of HIV seropositivity[8] and HIV seroconversion[24] among heroin addicts.

Cocaine use by methadone patients has many serious anti-therapeutic consequences. Kosten et al.'s follow-up of admissions to methadone treatment found that social adjustment deteriorated substantially with the onset of cocaine use and improved substantially with its cessation; cocaine abuse was associated with a relatively global deterioration in these subjects' functioning.[25] Black et al. reported that cocaine as well as cocaine combined with opiates contributed most frequently to failure on methadone maintenance and to the violation of contingency contracts.[26] The presence of active drug users in a methadone clinic also affects the morale of the compliant patients and of the staff.[27] Compliant patients resent being associated with active addicts who may approach them to buy or sell drugs. Staff may be frustrated because of their inability to help unstable patients and may believe that more motivated applicants are being denied scarce treatment slots. Increased crime[28] and increased diversion of methadone to the street,[29] are further consequences of cocaine use by methadone patients.

Few studies have examined changes in cocaine use after entry to methadone treatment. Chaisson et al. surveyed patients currently enrolled in methadone maintenance or detoxification in San Francisco.[8] Of those patients who reported ever using cocaine, 64% stopped or decreased cocaine use after entering treatment, 24% began or increased cocaine use, and 12% reported no change. It is not clear from this retrospective study, however, whether the changes reported pertain to the time of admission, the time of the survey, or refer to an average perceived change for the entire period of treatment. Correlates or predictors of changes in cocaine use also were not examined.

There have been only two prospective studies of cocaine use by addicts who were admitted to methadone treatment. Among a national sample of admissions to methadone treatment who remained at least 3 months, 26% used cocaine regularly in the year before treatment but only 9% were using regularly after 3 months of treatment; "regular use" was defined as once a week or more.[5] In addition, 18% of those who had left treatment were using cocaine regularly at a 1-year post-treatment follow-up, still a reduction from the pre-treatment level.

A 2 1/2 year follow-up of subjects who originally entered methadone treatment in 1979-80 found that 47% increased cocaine use, 25% decreased use, and 28% never used cocaine during the follow-up period.[30] However, only 29% of the methadone-treated subjects were still in a program at the time of follow-up, and separate rates of cocaine use for those remaining in treatment vs. those exiting from treatment were not given. Questions of how cocaine use changed after admission to treatment, and after exit from treatment, were not specifically examined by the study.

The results of these three studies of changes in cocaine use for addicts after entry to methadone treatment, taken at their face, could be considered inconsistent. Contributing to the problem of interpretation is that none of the studies employed a biological test for drug use (e.g., urinalysis) to help verify subjects' self-reports concerning cocaine use.[14] The two prospective studies also are based on ten year old admission cohorts, before the marked increase of general societal cocaine use during the 1980's and particularly before the introduction of crack in 1984-85 in the inner cities. The present study examines a more recent sample of admissions to methadone treatment (during 1987) and employs research urinalysis as a measure of cocaine use in addition to subjects' self-reports. The study seeks to address the following questions. What happens to addicts' cocaine use after entering methadone treatment? Although the rate of cocaine use among methadone patients is relatively high, do some addicts cease or decrease their use after admission, and do others begin or increase use? Finally, what characteristics of addicts at admission might predict changes in cocaine use after program entry?

METHODS

The study sample consists of 93 individuals admitted during 1987 to four methadone maintenance clinics in New York City (three in Manhattan, one in the Bronx). The subjects were interviewed within 30 days of admission, the majority within the first three days. Transfers from other methadone or treatment programs or any institutional setting were excluded; the intent was to include only individuals coming "off the street." The study interviewed 75% of the consecutive admissions during a three month data collection period at each clinic. Prospective subjects were informed that the research was studying problems that patients have in methadone maintenance and that the results could lead to treatment improvement. Participation in the study was voluntary and written informed consent was obtained. It was emphasized to subjects that the research was independent of the methadone clinic and that no individual interview or testing information would be available to clinic staff.

The subjects participated in 90-minute personal interviews and provided a urine specimen to researchers on the day of the interview. Follow-up interviews and urine specimens were obtained with 69% (N = 64) of the subjects between ten and eleven months after admission (termed the "one year follow-up"). All but one of the subjects who remained in the program were reinterviewed. For subjects who had left the program, data from clinic records and counselors were obtained to determine the circumstances of their departure. Subjects were paid an incentive of $30 at each data collection time. The interviews were conducted by trained paraprofessional interviewers who themselves were persons in recovery. Sociodemographic and treatment background characteristics of the study sample are given in Table 1.

The research urines were analyzed by enzyme multiplied immunoassay technique (EMIT) for cocaine and opiates. The EMIT cocaine test detects benzoylecgonine (the major metabolite of cocaine) at a concentration of 1.0 mcg/ml. The EMIT opiate test detects morphine, morphine glucuronide (the major metabolite of

Table 1: Sample Characteristics at Admission to Methadone Program (N = 93, in percent)

Gender		Employment Status	
Male	69	Full-time	9
Female	31	Part-time	5
Ethnicity		Unemployed*	84
Hispanic	58	In school	2
White	28	Previous Drug Abuse Treatment	
Black	14	Methadone maintenance	56
Age (In Years)		Residential drug-free	36
24 and under	13	Drug counseling	26
25 - 29	23	Narcotics/Cocaine Anonymous	31
30 - 34	30	Previous Mental Health Treatment	
35 - 39	18		
40 and over	16	Psychiatric hospitalization	14
Marital Status		Outpatient counseling only	13
Single, never married	45	Education	
Married	21	Less than high school	55
Separated/divorced	34	High school graduate	33
		Some college	12

* Of the unemployed, 26% (20/78) report performing some work "off the books" and 38% (30/78) are receiving public assistance.

heroin) and codeine, at minimum morphine-equivalent concentrations of 0.3 mcg/ml.[31]

Composite attitudinal and psychological scales were constructed based on factor analysis of several sets of fixed-response items on the interviews (principal factoring, varimax rotation). The scales were developed by the authors during a previous study using a cross-sectional sample of 285 methadone maintenance patients from the same participating programs.[32]

RESULTS

Cocaine Use at Admission to Methadone Treatment

Subjects were classified as current cocaine users if there was indication of use within 30 days before admission. The indicators were a cocaine-positive research urine taken no later than three days after admission or self-reported cocaine use during the month prior to admission. According to these criteria, 84% of the addicts entering methadone treatment were current cocaine users, in addition to using heroin (see Table 2). Table 2 also indicates that 97% of the sample has used cocaine at times in the past, that most have long histories of cocaine use, and that several routes of administration commonly are employed.

Changes in Cocaine Use Between Admission and Follow-up

Each patient's cocaine usage and program status were determined at follow-up, which was defined as about one year after admission for those still in program (70%) or at the time of discharge for those who had exited (30%) before one year. Outcome data were obtained from research interviews, research urinalysis, program records (including clinic urinalysis) and counselors for patients who remained, and only from program records and counselors for patients who had exited. A subject was classified as a cocaine user at follow-up if either the research data or program records indicated any cocaine use during the 30 days preceding the interview or exit from the program.

Table 2: Cocaine Use History (In percent)

Ever Used Cocaine		Length of Cocaine Use (Years)	
Cocaine (any kind)	97	1 - 5	12
Crack/freebase	59	6 - 10	36
Speedball	80	11 - 15	20
(N)	(93)	16 - 20	22
Age First Cocaine Use (Years)		20 and over	10
16 or under	33	(N)	(90)
17 - 19	22	Cocaine Use - Previous 30 Days Before Admission*	
20 - 24	23	No cocaine	16
25 - 29	15	Intranasal	16
30 and over	7	Injecting cocaine by itself	40
(N)	(90)	Crack/freebase	27
		Speedballing**	65
		(N)	(93)

*More than one route of administration may be stated.

** Injecting heroin and cocaine together.

Table 3 shows that 26% of the 78 subjects who had been using cocaine at admission were no longer using the drug at follow-up. Conversely, 20% of cocaine-free patients at admission reverted to cocaine use at follow-up (all had previous experience with cocaine). Because almost all of the sample were cocaine users at admission, this yields a net reduction of cocaine users from 84% at admission to 66% at follow-up. Among patients continuing to use cocaine at follow-up, there was a reduction in the reported mean number of days cocaine was ingested per month (from 16 to 9 days per month, $p < .01$, paired t-test), but not in the amount ingested per day of use.

Table 3: Changes in Cocaine Use Between Admission and Follow-up

	At Admission to Treatment			
	Cocaine Use		Cocaine - Free	
At Follow-up	%	(N)	%	(N)
Cocaine Use	74	(58)	20	(3)
Cocaine - Free	26	(20)	80	(12)
	100	(78)	100	(15)

Program Status and Cocaine Use at Follow-up

Patients who were using cocaine at admission tended to have a higher rate of program exit within one year than patients who were cocaine-free (33% vs. 13%), although this 20% difference does not reach statistical significance because of the small number (N = 15) of cocaine-free persons at admission. The reasons for exit were: administrative discharge for violations (42%), loss of contact (27%), incarceration (23%), and voluntary transfer or detoxification (8%). The rates of exit for patients using vs. not using cocaine at follow-up were similar (33% vs. 25%, n.s.). However, the reasons for exit were different in the two groups, with cocaine users accounting for all of the administrative discharges. It should be noted that cocaine use was rarely the sole reason for discharge; in fact most program staff believed it was better to retain cocaine-using patients in treatment whenever possible, since many had eliminated or reduced their heroin use.

Changes in Heroin Use and Intravenous Drug Use

All subjects were heroin injectors at the time they were admitted to the program. Among the patients who remained in their methadone program and were interviewed at follow-up, 59% (38/64) had negative research urines for opiates and said they had not used heroin within at least the preceding 30 days. Similarly, 61% (39/64) reported not injecting any drugs within the preceding 30 days. Indeed, almost all these individuals reported not injecting drugs or using heroin since their early days on the program. (These heroin use reports are also consistent with clinic urinalysis profiles over study period.) Among those continuing to inject drugs at follow-up (heroin and/or cocaine), the reported mean number of days of drug injection per month dropped from 24 to 12 days per month ($p < .001$, paired t-test).

Predictors of Change in Cocaine Use During Treatment

The ability to predict which patients are likely to continue cocaine use during treatment could assist in directing scarce services to the highest risk patients and in identifying the kinds of additional treatment or services needed. The study tried to determine which baseline variables might predict continuance/cessation of cocaine use at follow-up among those patients using cocaine at admission ($N = 78$). Baseline variables associated ($p < .05$) with continuing cocaine use at follow-up were: Age ($r = .24$), cocaine use before a previous treatment episode ($r = .28$), speedballing (injecting heroin and cocaine simultaneously) at current admission ($r = .28$), not sniffing cocaine at current admission ($r = -.26$), reports using cocaine for stimulation ($r = .24$), reports symptoms of depression ($r = .31$), low level of self-esteem ($r = -.31$), and seeks help for cocaine abuse at admission ($r = .25$). No other background or baseline variables correlated with continuing cocaine use at follow-up. Non-significant variables included: other sociodemographic variables, age of onset of cocaine use, other types/routes of cocaine use, other prior treatment experiences, other reported reasons for cocaine use such as pleasure or stress relief, perceived consequences of cocaine use, positive/negative attitudes towards cocaine use, prior attempts to abstain from cocaine, reported psychological symptoms, reported physical symptoms, and reported fatigue symptoms.

Baseline variables significantly correlated with continuance of cocaine use were entered as independent variables into a multiple logistic regression analysis (see Table 4). The results indicated that

Table 4: Stepwise Logistic Regression on Continuance of Cocaine Use at Follow-up
(N = 78)

	Adjusted Odds Ratio	Probability
Depressive Symptoms at Admission	1.17	.002
Speedballing at Admission	2.67	.005
Constant	.17	

Variables with F-values too small to enter the equation (p > .05) were: Age, Uses Cocaine for Stimulation, Seeks Help for Cocaine Use, Cocaine Use Before Previous Treatment Episode. Excluded from the regression because of high correlations (r > .7) with some other independent variables were: Self Esteem and Sniffing Cocaine at Admission.

two variables, reported symptoms of depression and speedballing at admission, explain significant amounts of variance in cocaine use at follow-up. (Depressive Symptoms was a 9-item scale derived from factor analysis with an internal consistency of alpha = .87.)

Program Services and Cocaine Use

Several programs in the study had ongoing "cocaine groups" led by counselors that cocaine-abusing patients sometimes were required to attend. About 8-12 patients in each program were enrolled at any given time. Among the patients interviewed at follow-up, only 7 had attended a cocaine group. However, 27 had attended one or more clinic groups of some kind, variously identified as "therapy," "education," "orientation," "AIDS awareness," etc., groups. Forty-four percent of those who attended such groups were cocaine-free at follow-up versus only 27% of those who did not attend any groups; but the difference was not statistically significant. Patients who were cocaine-free at follow-up were more likely to agree that being in the program had "helped them a lot" than patients who continued to use cocaine (86% vs. 62%, respectively, p < .05).

DISCUSSION

The very high rate of cocaine use (84%) among this methadone treatment admission cohort suggests that the "pure" heroin user has all but vanished from New York City. In fact, this rate is considerably higher than found in any previous study. The extensive cocaine-using history of the cohort is a clear signal that methadone maintenance programs must be prepared to treat cocaine as well as heroin addiction. This will require additional therapeutic tools, however, and primary cocaine treatment strategies unfortunately are still in an early stage of development.[33-36] Adequate funding would also be required to incorporate suitable cocaine treatment techniques into methadone programs.

One encouraging factor is that entry into methadone treatment does appear to reduce cocaine use in addition to most heroin use. Since this is occurring despite the unavailability of specialized cocaine treatment, one can suggest that providing state-of-the-art cocaine treatment — psychological, behavioral and/or pharmacological — might enhance the beneficial impact of entering a methadone program for persons dually addicted to heroin and cocaine.

As to why some cessation/reduction in cocaine use occurs, the interviews indicated that entry to methadone treatment is generally stabilizing for many addicts, so that there is less desire or pressure to "hustle" for any drugs. Moreover, many addicts entering treatment have "hit bottom" and state a strong motivation to eliminate all "hard" drug use, which some apparently are able to achieve with the assistance of a substitute opiate and a supportive program environment. That cocaine-free individuals were somewhat more likely to have participated in clinic group activities suggests the importance of a therapeutic environment, although of course group participants were self-selected and probably more disposed to accepting help.

This prospective study identified the level of depressive symptoms at admission as a significant predictor of continued cocaine use during treatment. In addition, 50% of the patients reported specifically that their cocaine use increases when they feel "down" (i.e., depressed). It has been observed that self-regulation of painful emotions is an important factor in drug abuse in general.[37] Previous studies have documented that many addicts admitted to methadone treatment suffer from episodic or chronic depression.[16,38] However, whether depression is a cause or consequence (or both) of drug use has remained unclear. The evidence of this study is that depression, whether clinical or situational, is an important antecedent of cocaine use and not solely the result of habitual use. Nevertheless, users appear to understand the vicious cycle inherent in chronic cocaine use, since 82% of the patients also agreed that "after using coke, I feel lower than before." (Low self-esteem, which was strongly related to depressive symptoms, may also account for some continuing cocaine use in this cohort.) These findings support the use of appropriate pharmacotherapies (e.g., tricyclic antidepressants) for clinically depressed patients[39,40] as well as cognitive therapies that have shown utility with depressed individuals,[41] if suitably modified for a substance-abusing population.

REFERENCES

1. Abdul-Quader AS, Friedman SR, Des Jarlais D, Marmor MM, Maslansky R, and Bartelme S. Methadone maintenance and behavior by intravenous drug users that can transmit HIV. Contemporary Drug Problems 1987:425-434.

2. Anglin MD, McGlothlin WH. Outcome of narcotic addict treatment in California. In: Tims F and Ludford J, eds. Drug abuse treatment evaluation: strategies, progress and prospects. NIDA Research Monograph 51. Washington DC: US Government Printing Office, 1984: 106-128.

3. Ball JC, Lange RW, Myers PC, Friedman SR. Reducing the risk of AIDS through methadone treatment. Journal of Health and Social Behavior 1988; 29: 214-226.

4. Hubbard RL, Marsden ME, Cavanaugh E, Rachal JV, Ginzburg HM. Role of drug abuse treatment in limiting the spread of AIDS. Reviews of Infectious Diseases 1988: 10: 377-384.

5. Hubbard RL, Marsden ME, Rachal JV, Harwood HJ, Cavanaugh ER, Ginzburg HM. Drug abuse treatment: a national study of effectiveness. Chapel Hill, NC: University of North Carolina Press, 1989.

6. Simpson DD, Sells SB. Effectiveness of treatment for drug abuse: An overview of the DARP research program. Advances in Alcohol & Substance Abuse 1982; 2: 7-29.

7. Marmor M, Des Jarlais DC, Cohen H, Friedman SR, Beatrice ST, Dubin N, El-Sadr W, Mildvan D, Yancovitz S, Mathur U, Holzman R. Risk factors for infection with human immunodeficiency virus among intravenous drug abusers in New York City. AIDS 1987; 1: 39-44.

8. Chaisson RE, Bacchetti P, Osmong E, Brodie B, Sande M and Moss A.

Cocaine use and HIV infection in intravenous drug users in San Francisco. Journal of the American Medical Association 1989; 261: 561-565.

9. Blix O, Gronbladh L. AIDS and IV heroin addicts: The preventive effect of methadone maintenance in Sweden. Proceedings of the Fourth International Conference on AIDS. Stockholm, 1988.

10. Hartel D, Schoenbaum EE, Selwyn PA, Drucker E, Wasserman W, Friedland GW. Temporal patterns of cocaine use and AIDS in intravenous drug users in methadone maintenance. Proceedings of the Fifth International Conference on AIDS. Montreal, 1989.

11. Novick DM, Joseph H, Richman BL, Salsitz EA, Pascarelli EF, Des Jarlais DC, Dole VP. Medical maintenance: A new model for continuing treatment of socially rehabilitated methadone maintenance patients. In: Harris LS, ed. Problems of drug dependence, 1988. NIDA Research Monograph. Washington, DC: Government Printing Office, 1989.

12. Truman B, Lehman JS, Brown L, Peyser N, Peters D, Des Jarlais D. HIV infection among intravenous drug users in NYC. Proceedings of the Fifth International Conference on AIDS, Montreal, 1989.

13. Strug DL, Hunt DE, Goldsmith DS, Lipton DS and Spunt B. Patterns of cocaine use among methadone clients. International Journal of the Addictions 1985; 20:1163-1175.

14. Magura S, Goldsmith D, Casriel C, Goldstein PJ, Lipton DS. The validity of methadone clients' self-reported drug use. International Journal of the Addictions 1987; 22:727-749.

15. Hanbury R, Sturiano V, Cohen M, Stimmel B, Aguillaume C. Cocaine use in persons on methadone maintenance. Advances in Alcohol & Substance Abuse 1987; 6: 97-106.

16. Corty E, Ball JC. Admissions to methadone maintenance: comparisons between programs and implications for treatment. Journal of Substance Abuse Treatment 1987; 4: 181-187.

17. Division of Substance Abuse Services. Program statistics. Albany, NY: New York State Division of Substance Abuse Services, 1990.

18. General Accounting Office. Preliminary findings: a survey of methadone maintenance programs. Washington, DC: General Accounting Office, 1989.

19. Kerr P. Cocaine use up among methadone patients. New York Times 1986; October 12: 43.

20. Landis B. Hooked—the madness in methadone maintenance. Village Voice 1988; April 5: 31.

21. New York Newsday. Cashing in on methadone. New York Newsday 1989; June 4: 6.

22. National Institute on Drug Abuse. NIDA outreach demonstration projects provide insight into AIDS risk behaviors. NIDA Notes 1989; 4: 1-9.

23. Magura S, Grossman JI, Lipton DS, Siddiqi Q, Shapiro J, Marion I, Amann KR. Determinants of needle sharing among intravenous drug users. American Journal of Public Health 1989; 79: 459-462.

24. Des Jarlais, DC and Friedman, SR. Intravenous cocaine, crack, and HIV

infection. Journal of the American Medical Association, Letter to the Editor, 1988; 259: 1945-1946.

25. Kosten TR, Rounsaville BJ, Kleber HD. Antecedents and consequences of cocaine abuse among opioid addicts. Journal of Nervous and Mental Disease 1988; 176: 176-181.

26. Black JL, Dolan MP, Penk WE, Robinowitz R, DeFord HA. The effect of increased cocaine use on drug treatment. Addictive Behaviors 1987; 12: 289-292.

27. Hunt DE, Strug DL, Goldsmith DS, Lipton DS, Spunt BJ, Truitt L, Robertson KA. An instant shot of 'Aah': cocaine use among methadone clients. Journal of Psychoactive Drugs 1984; 16: 217-227.

28. Hunt DE, Lipton DS, Spunt B. Patterns of criminal activity among methadone clients and current narcotics users not in treatment. Journal of Drug Issues 1984; 14: 687-702.

29. Spunt B, Hunt DE, Lipton DS, Goldsmith DS. Methadone diversion: A new look. Journal of Drug Issues 1986; 16: 569-583.

30. Kosten TR, Rounsaville BJ, Kleber HD. A 2.5 year follow-up of cocaine abuse among opiate addicts. Have our treatments helped? Archives of General Psychiatry 1987; 44: 281-285.

31. SYVA Company. Emit® d.a.u. tests for drugs of abuse in urine. Palo Alto, CA: SYVA, 1983.

32. Magura S, Siddiqi Q, Freeman RC, Lipton DS. Cocaine use and help-seeking among methadone patients. Journal of Drug Issues 1991; 21: 629-645.

33. Washton, AM. Structured outpatient treatment of cocaine abuse. Advances in Alcohol & Substance Abuse 1987; 143-157.

34. Wallace BC. Relapse prevention in psychoeducational groups for compulsive crack cocaine smokers. Journal of Substance Abuse Treatment 1989; 6: 229-239.

35. Matrix Center. The neurobehavioral treatment model. Beverly Hills, CA: Matrix Center, Inc., 1989.

36. Gawin FH, Ellinwood EH. Cocaine and other stimulants: actions, abuse and treatment. New England Journal of Medicine 1988; 318: 1173-1182.

37. Khantzian EJ. Self-selection and progression in drug dependence. In: Shaffer H and Burglass ME, eds. Classic contributions in the addictions. New York: Brunner/Mazel, 1981: 154-60.

38. Rounsaville BJ, Weissman MM, Kleber H, Wilber C. Heterogeneity of psychiatric diagnosis in treated opiate addicts. Archives of General Psychiatry 1982; 39:161-6.

39. O'Brien CP, Childress AR, Arndt IO, McLellan AT, Woody GE, Maany I. Pharmacological and behavioral treatments of cocaine dependence: controlled studies. Journal of Clinical Psychiatry 1988; 49 (2, suppl): 17-22.

40. Kosten TR, Schumann RN, Wright D, Carney MK, Gawin FH. A preliminary study of desipramine in the treatment of cocaine abuse in methadone maintenance patients. Journal of Clinical Psychiatry 1987; 48: 442-444.

41. Beck AT, Rush AJ, Shaw BF, Emery G. Cognitive therapy of depression. New York: Guilford, 1979.

Cardiovascular Evaluation After Withdrawal from Chronic Alcohol or Cocaine-Alcohol Abuse

Ralph M. Moskowitz, MD
Anthony J. Errichetti, MD

SUMMARY. Alcohol ingestion commonly accompanies cocaine abuse, but the effects of chronic cocaine-alcohol abuse on the circulation are undefined. Therefore, to test for evidence of cocaine-alcohol cardiac dysfunction and interference with cardiovascular nervous system reflexes, 10 normal volunteers (group I), 8 asymptomatic alcoholic patients (group II), and 15 age matched, asymptomatic cocaine and alcohol abusers (group III) underwent screening two-dimensional echocardiography, electrocardiography, a series of autonomic nervous system tests, and upright bicycle exercises. Echocardiographic indices did not differ among groups. R wave voltage was increased in group III, probably primarily due to a smaller body surface area. Heart rate (HR) and/or systolic blood pressure (SBP) responses to 60 degree tilt and to hyperventilation differed in group III (decreased HR response, while SBP increased inappropriately). Despite excellent exercise tolerance, HR response to exercise in group III (compared to group I) was decreased. These results suggest impairment of certain autonomic nervous system re-

Ralph M. Moskowitz and Anthony J. Errichetti are affiliated with the Cardiology Section, Medical Service, and the Psychiatry Service, Martinez Veterans Affairs Medical Center and the Departments of Medicine and Psychiatry, University of California, Davis.

Technical assistance was provided by Joyce M. Michelson, MS, RN and Joann Dandurand, RN.

Requests for reprints should be addressed to Ralph Moskowitz, MD, Cardiology Section (111B), Martinez VA Medical Center, 150 Muir Road, Martinez, CA 94553.

flexes and, possibly, sinus node dysfunction from cocaine-alcohol abuse.

INTRODUCTION

Since 1980 an epidemic of cocaine abuse has occurred in the United States.[1] However, use of cocaine alone is relatively infrequent; a large majority of cocaine abusers also abuse other psychoactive agents, most commonly alcohol.[2] In this regard, though the clinicopathological features of alcoholic cardiomyopathy are well described,[3-4] evidence for cocaine-induced cardiac dysfunction is less well defined;[5-8] similarly, the occurrence of circulatory abnormalities among chronic cocaine-alcohol abusers is unclear. Also, evidence of autonomic dysfunction with increased sympathetic tone is frequently found in patients after withdrawal from chronic alcoholism,[9-10] but despite some animal data suggesting catecholamine depletion after prolonged cocaine administration,[11] little is known about the chronic effects of cocaine or cocaine and alcohol on the autonomic nervous system.[12] Therefore, in order to compare the effects of long-term alcohol and cocaine-alcohol exposure on cardiac function and cardiovascular reflexes in humans, we performed screening electrocardiography and two-dimensional echocardiography at rest, upright bicycle exercise, and several tests of autonomic nervous system function in (1) normal control subjects; (2) asymptomatic patients recently withdrawn from chronic ethanolism; and (3) asymptomatic patients recently withdrawn from chronic cocaine and ethanol abuse. The results indicate differences in heart rate (HR) and blood pressure responses among these three groups.

SUBJECTS AND METHODS

Patients: Ten healthy control males (group I), eight male alcoholics (group II), and fifteen cocaine and alcohol abusers (group III) were studied. Study patients were selected in sequence from all patients admitted to the alcohol and drug abuse treatment program at the Martinez VA Medical Center. The hospital's human studies subcommittee approved the investigation and all subjects gave written informed consent. Criteria for exclusion included prior heart disease, symptoms of unusual dyspnea on exertion, orthopnea, or ankle swelling, valvular abnormalities on a screening two-dimensional Doppler echocardiogram, ischemic ST segment depression during exercise, prior or current hypertension (greater than 160/90 mm Hg) lasting beyond three days after admission, diabetes mellitus, anemia, thyroid disorders, significant pulmonary or renal disease, atrial fibrillation, treatment with cardiovascular medications, and inability to perform bicycle exercise. Patients admitting to recent drug use (other than cocaine or marijuana) were also excluded. A routine urine sample obtained at the time of admission to the hospital was analyzed for amphetamines, cocaine, cannabis, opiates, and ethanol.

Group I subjects drank 18 or less g of ethanol daily, denied drug use, and had negative urinary drug and ethanol screens; two persons in group I smoked cigarettes regularly and one was a former smoker. Each group II patient consumed at least 80 g of alcohol per day for a mean period of 12.9 years (range three to twenty-one years); one group II patient gave a history of marijuana use every two days (last exposure two days prior to study) and had a positive urinary screen for cannabinoids; the remaining group II patients gave no history of drug use and had negative urinary screening tests. Six group II patients smoked cigarettes regularly. Eight group III subjects drank at least 80 g of ethanol per day for an average of 13.9 years (range 4-20 years); these eight patients also used cocaine daily or several times per week for a mean of 7.8 years (range 4-15 years). The remaining group III patients drank 40-80 g of ethanol per day, and had a history of cocaine abuse over a mean of 5.6 years (range 0.5-19 years). Urine screens for cocaine were positive in 13 group III patients. Seven group III subjects gave history of marijuana use. Of these, two admitted to occasional use (1-2 times per month) and had positive urine tests for cannabinoids (last use by each patient 2 and 5 days prior to study respectively). Among the other five, one patient smoked one joint per day almost daily in the last month, two patients smoked one or more joints per day, and one patient smoked one joint two days per week; urine screening for cannabinoids was positive in one of the five patients tested (last exposure in this patient 2 days prior to study). No other group III patient had a positive urine test for cannabinoids. Seven group III patients were cigarette smokers. All subjects had normal cardiovascular physical examination results. No patient had hepatomegaly, ascites, jaundice, or other physical signs of chronic liver disease. Two group II patients had elevations of serum liver function tests which reverted toward normal on repeat testing; four group III patients showed minimally elevated liver function tests which were not retested.

Group II patients were studied at a mean of 3.7 days (range 2-5 days) after abstinence. Group III patients were studied 5.4 days (range 2-14 days) after last cocaine use, and 3.8 days (range 2-7 days) after withdrawal from ethanol. All subjects were studied in the morning beginning one hour after a clear liquid breakfast. A supine 12-lead electrocardiogram was obtained and two-dimensional Doppler and M-mode echocardiography were performed in all subjects. M-mode measurements were made in a standard manner.[13] Left ventricular dimensions could not be measured in one patient because of inadequate recording quality. Height and weight were measured and body surface area was calculated based on the Dubois and Dubois height-weight equation. HR during each intervention was obtained by electrocardiographic recording over a 15-20 second period; cuff systolic blood pressure (SBP) and diastolic blood pressure (DBP) was obtained by oscillometry (DINAMAP) or (during hyperventilation and exercise) by mercury syphgmomanometry. The following tests were performed in sequence with fifteen minutes of recovery between evaluations: (1) Tilt-table: subjects were supine for fifteen minutes and then tilted 60 degrees for twenty minutes; hemodynamics were measured supine, 1 minute upright, 5 minutes upright, and then at 5 minute intervals; (2) Cold-pressor test: while supine, the hand was immersed in ice-water for two minutes; hemodynamics were recorded at baseline, at two minutes cold exposure, and after two minutes of recovery; (3) Mental arithmetic: while supine, subjects performed five minutes of mental arithmetic; hemodynamics were obtained at rest and at one minute intervals; (4) Hyperventilation: while sitting, subjects hyperventilated for three minutes; hemodynamics were obtained before and at each minute of testing; (5) Bicycle exercise: after sitting upright for fifteen minutes, subjects underwent symptom limited exercise on a bicycle ergometer; workload was increased by 25 watts every three minutes while pedal speed was kept at 60 revolutions per minute; hemodynamics were obtained at rest and during the third minute of each successive stage.

Statistical Methods:[14-15] Grouped data are expressed as mean ± SEM. The effect of a given test (other than exercise) among the groups over the entire period of the test was evaluated by one factor analysis of variance for repeated measures. A difference among the groups at one point in time was assessed by one factor analysis of variance. If analyses of variance revealed a statistically significant difference, intergroup comparisons were performed using the Scheffe test. Exercise results in group I and group III at each workload were compared using the Student's t-test for unpaired data. Regression lines for the cumulated effect of exercise upon HR, SBP, DBP and the double product of SBP × HR were obtained using the least squares technique and compared by repeated measures analysis of variance with an orthogonal polynomial decomposition. P values less than 0.05 were considered statistically significant.

RESULTS

Mean age in group I subjects was 36.2 ± 2.1 years (range 24-45), 36.8 ± 2.5 years (range 25-43) in group II, and 31.9 ± 1.5 years (range 23-44) years in group III (p = NS).

Height, weight, and body surface area (Table 1): Mean height and weight did not show any statistically significant differences among groups (p = NS). Mean body surface area, however, differed among groups ($p < 0.05$). Intergroup comparisons revealed a significant statistical difference between group I and group III ($p < 0.05$).

Echocardiography (Table 2): There were no significant differences with respect to left ventricular wall thickness, chamber size, E point septal separation, fractional shortening, or left atrial and aortic root size among the three groups.

Electrocardiography (Table 3): There were no statistically significant differences among groups with respect to rate, frontal plane R

TABLE 1. Height, Weight, and Body Surface Area in Groups I, II, and III

Parameter	Group I	Group II	Group III	p-value
Height	71.1 ±.9	70.4 ±.6	69.9 ±.6	p=NS
Weight	190 ± 8	175 ± 5	170 ± 5	"
BSA	2.1 ± .05	2.0 ± .02	1.9 ±.03	p<.05

Heights are in inches; weights are in pounds; body surface area (BSA) in square meters. Values are mean ± standard error of the mean.

wave axis, P wave axis, T wave axis, QRS duration, PR interval, or QTc. A statistically significant increase in R wave voltage among group III patients was seen in frontal plane leads 2 and AVF, as well as precordial leads V1 and V5.

Tilt-table (Table 4, Fig 1): Mean supine SBP did not differ among groups (p = NS). During tilt, however, mean SBP decreased in group I, increased slightly in group II, and increased more so in group III. Average SBP during the 20 min. was 120.7 ± 1.9 mm Hg for group I, 120.5 ± 1.6 for group II, and 131.7 ± 1.5 for group III (p < 0.03). After the initial minute of tilt, mean change in SBP from supine was in group I -5.5 ± 4.1, in group II -0.8 ± 4.8, and in group III 6.6 ± 1.6 (p < 0.03); group I and group III differed significantly (p < 0.04). Mean supine DBP did not differ significantly among groups; during tilt, mean DBP rose in each group, without differences among groups being present.

Mean supine HR did not differ among groups (n = NS). During tilt, mean HR in group I was 77.9 ± 1.2, group II 82.8 ± 1.3, and in group III 72.7 ± 1.2 (p < 0.04). Group II and group III differed significantly (p < 0.05). At one minute of tilt, mean change in HR in group I was 17.9 ± 1.9, in group II 14.5 ± 2.2, and in group III 7.9 ± 1.4 (p < 0.0005); group III differed from both group I and group II (p < 0.0005 and p < 0.04, respectively).

Cold pressor test (Table 4): There were no statistically significant

TABLE 2. Echocardiographic Values in Groups I, II, and III

Parameter	Group I	Group II	Group III
PW	9.3 ± .3	9.3 ± .6	9.7 ± .3
IVS	9.4 ± .4	10.0 ± .5	9.9 ± .2
LVEDD	49.3 ± 1.2	48.7 ± 2.1	60.7 ± 1.7
LVESD	32.5 ± 1.1	31.9 ± 1.4	33.5 ± 1.7
EPSS	1.9 ± .8	2.9 ± .9	3.9 ± .8
FS	0.33 ± .02	0.36 ± .01	0.34 ± .02
LA	34.6 ± 1.6	33.1 ± 1.8	34.6 ± 1.1
AR	34.2 ± .8	33.0 ± 1.3	32.3 ± .6

Dimensions are given in mm. Data are mean ± standard error of the mean. Abbreviations: AR = aortic root; EPSS = E point septal separation; FS = fractional shortening; IVS = intraventricular septal thickness; LA = left atrium; LVEDD left ventricular end-diastolic diameter; LVESD = left ventricular end-systolic diameter; PW = posterior wall thickness

differences in SBP or DBP among the groups at rest. During ice immersion, mean SBP and DBP rose in each group, without differences among groups being present. Mean HR at rest in group II was elevated ($p < 0.01$). Mean HR during cold exposure did not show statistically significant differences among groups ($p = $ NS); also, mean change in HR from rest to ice immersion did not differ ($p = $ NS). Mean SBP and DBP at 2 minutes of recovery did not differ among groups ($p = $ NS). Similar to baseline values, mean HR during recovery in group II was raised ($p < 0.01$).

Mental stress (Table 5): There were no statistically significant

TABLE 3. Electrocardiographic Values in Groups I, II, and III

Parameter	Group I	Group II	Group III	p-value
R wave axis	52.0 ± 8.3	47.4 ± 13.0	70.3 ± 2.5	p=NS
T wave axis	38.0 ± 6.8	38.7 ± 10.0	45.4 ± 5.5	"
P wave axis	44.3 ± 9.3	27.4 ± 13.3	45.7 ± 5.7	"
PR interval	163 ± 5.1	146 ± 8.3	165 ± 4.4	"
QRS interval	96 ± 2.2	98 ± 2.7	95 ± 3.0	"
QTc interval	398 ± 3.7	407 ± 5.3	401 ± 3.6	"
R wave volts:				
Lead 1	6.2 ± 1.2	7.0 ± 1.3	6.5 ± .5	"
Lead 2	8.1 ± 0.6	9.9 ± 1.6	+ * 18.4 ± 1.8	p<.0001
Lead AVL	3.3 ± 0.9	3.6 ± 1.2	1.4 ± 0.3	p=NS
Lead AVF	5.6 ± 0.7	7.3 ± 1.7	++ * 15.1 ± 1.7	p<.0005
Lead V1	1.7 ± 0.4	2.7 ± 0.3	+++ 3.3 ± 0.4	p<.05
Lead V3	9.4 ± 2.0	8.7 ± 1.1	11.2 ± 1.5	p=NS
Lead V5	16.4 ± 0.7	16.9 ± 1.7	** 22.2 ± 1.8	p<.025

Frontal plane axes are in degrees; intervals are in msec; voltages are in millivolts. Values are mean ± standard error of the mean. + = p<0.0005 Group I vs Group III. * = p<0.01 group II vs Group III. ++ = p<0.005 Group I vs Group III. +++ = p<0.05 Group I vs Group III. ** = p<0.025 Group I vs Group III.

differences in SBP or DBP among groups at rest or during 5 min. of mental arithmetic. However, mean HR at rest in group II was elevated (p < 0.025). There were no statistically significant differences during testing in mean HR among groups (p = NS). Change in HR during testing differed among groups (p < 0.04). Change in HR was less in group II than in group I (p < 0.05).

TABLE 4. Hemodynamic Responses to Tilt Table and Cold Pressor Testing in Groups I, II, and III

Test	Minutes	Systolic Blood Pressure				Heart Rate			
		Group I	Group II	Group III	p-value	Group I	Group II	Group III	p-value
		(n=10)	(n=8)	(n=15)		(n=10)	(n=8)	(n=15)	
Tilt Table	0	124.2±2.7	119 ±3.0	125.6±3.5	p=NS	60.3±1.9	67.6±4.3	62.1±2.3	p=NS
	1	119.5±3.9	117.1±4.2	132.3±3.2	p<.025	78.2±2.7	82.1±3.4	69.9±2.5	p<.025
	5	127.3±5.1	121.5±3.1	129.8±3.6	p=NS	78 ±2.5	82.5±3.2	71.4±2.9	p<.05
	10	119.3±3.9	119.6±3.3	132.5±3.0	p<.025	76.4±3.1	83.8±3.4	73.6±2.5	p=NS
	15	119.4±3.7	122.8±3.9	130.6±3.9	p=NS	78.4±2.7	83.9±2.8	73.6±2.7	p<.05
	20	120.6±4.8	120.4±3.4	133.5±3.4	p<.05	79 ±3.1	81.8±2.6	74.9±2.5	p=NS
Cold Pressor	0	120.7±4.2	121 ±5.6	126. ±3.7	p=NS	60.4±1.7	71.1±4.3	59.5±2.0	p<.01
	2	144.5±6.5	132.6±6.9	139.9±5.8	"	70.5±3.1	78.4±4.3	74.1±3.6	p=NS
	4	127.9±2.8	121. ±5.0	124.5±3.6	"	60.4±1.8	71. ±3.7	59.2±2.3	p<.01

Legend: Data are mean ± standard error of the mean.
Values in parentheses are the number in each group contributing to the mean;
p-values are results of one factor analysis of variance at individual minutes.

55

FIGURE 1. Relation between minutes of tilt to 60 degrees and systolic blood pressure (A) and heart rate (B) in Group I (n = 10), Group II (n = 8), and Group III (n = 15). Values are ± standard error of the mean. Statistical significance valuess refer to results of analysis of variance at individual times.

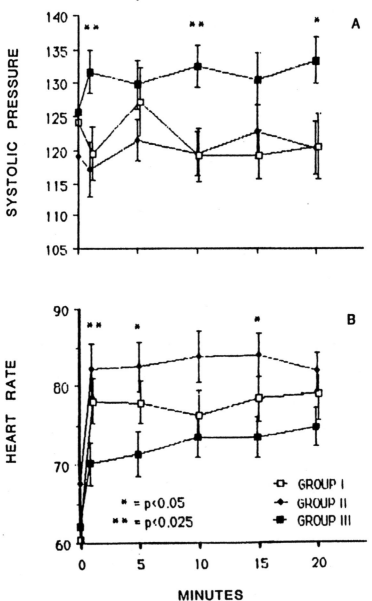

TABLE 5. Hemodynamic Responses to Mental Arithmetic and Hyperventilation in Groups I, II, and III

Test	Minutes	Systolic Blood Pressure				Heart Rate			
		Group I (n=9)	Group II (n=8)	Group III (n=15)	p-value	Group I (n=9)	Group II (n=8)	Group III (n=15)	p-value
Mental Arithmetic	0	123 ±3.5	124.9±4.3	122.1±3.2	p = NS	61.7±1.7	70.8±4.4	58.5±2.3	p < .025
	1	132.9±3.4	131.1±3.3	132.1±4.4	"	71.7±2.9	75.1±5.3	66.9±2.9	p = NS
	2	134.4±3.0	127.8±5.0	129.9±4.2	"	68.8±3.3	73.4±4.7	65.3±2.3	"
	3	130.2±4.2	129.4±5.4	127.1±4.2	"	70.2±2.7	74.4±4.5	65.9±2.3	"
	4	128.6±4.5	129.6±4.9	130.9±4.1	"	71.9±3.2	73.8±4.1	66.6±2.4	"
	5	132.1±4.1	125.8±6.5	127.1±3.5	"	73.4±3.2	74 ±4.3	66.1±2.3	"
Hyperventilation		(n=9)	(n=5)	(n=10)		(n=9)	(n=5)	(n=10)	
	0	114.1±2.6	115 ±1.3	121.6±4.0	p = NS	69.2±2.9	74.8±4.7	67.3±2.4	p = NS
	1	110.1±5.9	110.8±2.6	123.2±3.8	"	95.3±5.4	85.8±7.7	79.4±6.1	"
	2	107.8±5.6	109.6±3.5	123 ±3.5	"	93.6±6.0	94 ±7.9	79.8±4.5	"
	3	109 ±3.8	112 ±3.8	123.2±3.3	p < .025	93.4±5.6	94.8±8.1	81.8±3.7	"

Legend: Data are mean ± standard error of the mean.
Values in parentheses are the number of subject in each group contributing to the mean;
p-values are results of one factor analysis of variance at individual minutes.

Hyperventilation (Table 5, Fig 2): Mean SBP at rest did not differ statistically among groups. During hyperventilation mean SBP decreased in groups I and II to 108.8 ± 2.8 and 110.8 ± 1.9 respectively, and increased in group III to 123.2 ± 2.1 (p < 0.03). Intergroup comparisons revealed group I and group III to have a statistically significant difference (p < 0.04). Mean DBP did not differ significantly among groups at rest or during hyperventilation. Mean resting HR did not show a statistically significant difference among groups (p = NS). During 3 min. of testing mean HR was lower in group III (80.3 ± 2.7) than in group I (94.1 ± 3.2) or in group II (91.7 ± 4.5); these values almost showed a statistically significant difference among groups (p < 0.1).

Bicycle Exercise (Table 5, Fig 3): Mean exercise duration in group I was 23.1 ± 0.9 min, in group II 17.6 ± 1.8 min, and in group III 21.6 ± min (p < 0.05). Because of the decreased exercise tolerance among group II patients, group I and group III data were compared. Mean SDP and DBP prior to exercise did not differ significantly (p = NS for both). However, mean HR was lower in group II than in group I at rest (p < 0.01), as well as at each stage of exercise (Table 5). Regression analysis for HR data during stress in group I yielded the equation y = 0.451x + 66.6 (r = .92), and in group II, y = 0.434x + 60.0 (r = .91). Repeated measures analysis indicated that these regression lines had statistically significant different intercepts (p < 0.05). Mean SBP tended to be slightly higher in group III vs. group I during exercise (Table 5); however, repeated measures analysis of the calculated regression lines did not show statistical significance (p = NS). Similarly, the double product of HR multiplied by SBP (Table 5) tended to be higher in group I than group III during exercise, but comparison of regression lines did not reveal a statistically significant difference (p = NS). Mean DBP during exercise did not differ.

DISCUSSION

The acute administration of ethanol and cocaine to humans causes augmentation of HR beyond that seen with either agent by itself.[16] No information is available, however, concerning the

FIGURE 2. Relation between minutes of hyperventilation and systolic blood pressure (A) and heart rate (B) in Group I (n = 9), Group II (n = 5), and Group III (n = 10). Values are means ± sdtandard error of the mean. Statistical significance value refers to result of analysis of variance at individual time.

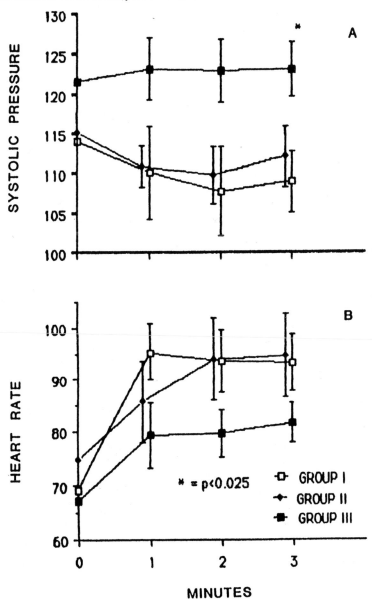

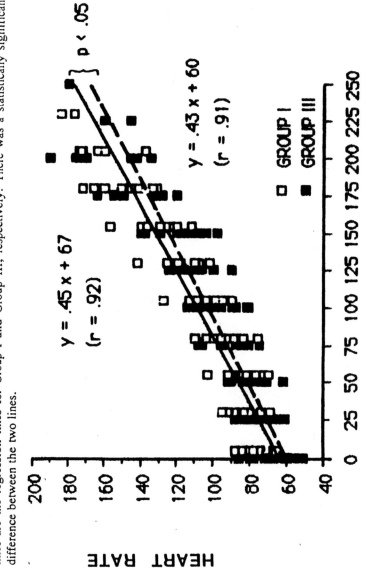

FIGURE 3. Relation between watts of bicycle exercise and heart rate in Group I and Group III. Solid and dashed lines are the regression lines for Group I and Group III, respectively. There was a statistically significant difference between the two lines.

60

chronic effects of these drugs in combination. The results of the present study reveal alterations among group III alcohol and cocaine abusers. Overall, cardiac pump function at rest (as evidenced by left ventricular dimensions and systolic function on echocardiography) and during exercise (as seen by exercise duration) appears normal. However, HR and/or SBP responses to tilt, hyperventilation, and exercise in group III show differences from group I control subjects and/or group II alcoholic patients: (1) during tilt, mean SBP rose, while mean HR (and change in HR at one minute) were less than the other groups; (2) during hyperventilation, mean SBP increased; (3) compared to normal subjects, while sitting upright prior to exercise, HR was decreased (a finding similar to the HR response after tilt); and (4) compared to normals, during exercise HR was decreased. These findings suggest a cocaine-alcohol related impairment of certain autonomic nervous system reflex blood pressure and chronotropic responses.

The increased HR (seen before ice immersion and mental arithmetic, as well as before and during tilt) in group II patients is consistent with prior data and is likely due to increased sympathetic tone[9-10] or parasympathetic impairment[17] present after alcohol withdrawal. Despite chronic exposure to ethanol, however, compared to group II alcoholic subjects, resting HR values and/or HR during stress (tilt, bicycle exercise) in group III patients were decreased (see Table 6). This suggests a predominant counterbalancing residual negative chronotropic effect of cocaine. Such an effect is consistent with evidence (from rats chronically given cocaine) of myocardial norepinephrine deletion and heart rate slowing,[12,18] while resting blood pressure was unaffected.[18] Adrenal and serum levels of catecholamines increase in rats chronically given cocaine,[18-19] but compared to controls, the atrial heart rate response to norepinephrine[20] or epinephrine[21] is decreased after treatment with repeated doses of cocaine. Avakian and coworkers hypothesized that decreased cardiac beta-receptor density or affinity might occur after cocaine exposure, but evaluation failed to document such alterations.[22]

Direct myocardial injury due to cocaine-alcohol abuse may also contribute to impairment of chronotropic function. Tissue obtained from endomyocardial biopsy specimens in alcoholic patients show

TABLE 6. Hemodynamic Responses to Bicycle Exercise in Group I and Group II.

Workload	Systolic Blood Pressure		Heart Rate		Double Product x 10^{-2}	
	Group I	Group III	Group I	Group III	Group I	Group III
0 W	116.7±3.5 (10)	118.7±3.5 (15)	75.4±2.4 (10)	65.8±2.6 (15)	87.8±3.0 (10)	78.9±4.8 (15)
25 W	121.3±2.7 (10)	122.3±2.8 (15)	82.4±2.6 (10)	75.5±2.1 (15)	99.7±3.0 (10)	91.4±3.8 (15)
50 W	124.9±2.6 (10)	123.5±3.4 (15)	85.7±3.1 (10)	80.8±2.2 (15)	107.1±4.7 (10)	91.0±6.5 (15)
75 W	128.1±3.0 (10)	132.5±3.9 (15)	93.7±3.2 (10)	88.1±2.4 (15)	118.5±4.9 (10)	114.5±4.1 (15)
100 W	138.8±3.5 (10)	135.2±3.4 (15)	105.6±3.4 (10)	97.4±2.5 (15)	147.6±6.3 (10)	131.4±4.0 (15)
125 W	146 ±3.0 (10)	150.1±3.6 (14)	118.3±3.5 (10)	109.4±2.8 (14)	172.8±6.6 (10)	164.6±6.4 (14)
150 W	159.6±4.0 (10)	167.6±4.0 (14)	131.2±4.0 (10)	119.5±3.5 (14)	209.0±9.8 (10)	198.7±8.1 (14)
175W	167.4±4.7 (9)	183.2±7.1 (8)	151.4±4.7 (9)	141.9±5.4 (8)	255.1±14.0 (9)	262.0±14.4 (8)
200 W	186.3±4.9 (6)	193.1±5.8 (7)	163.5±5.6 (6)	162.7±7.6 (7)	305.3±15.0 (6)	315.3±20.7 (7)
225 W	187.0±1.1 (2)	194.0±6.0 (2)	180.5±3.5 (2)	153.0±7.0 (2)	337.2±13.3 (2)	296.4±4.4 (2)
250 W	195 (1)		180 (1)		276 (1)	

Legend: Data are mean ± standard error of the mean. W = watts.
Values in parentheses are the number of patients contributing to the mean.

cardiomyopathyic changes.[4] Cocaine may damage the myocardium either by causing a toxic (due to local accumulation of excess catecholamine) or hypersensitivity myocarditis.[6-7] The occurrence of myocardial contraction bands and focal myocardial necrosis in hearts autopsied from human cocaine abusers,[5] as well as the appearance of necrosis and focal myocarditis in transvenous right ventricular endomyocardial biopsy specimens obtained from living cocaine abusers[7] suggest that long-term cocaine-alcohol exposure could lead to sinus node dysfunction.

The increased electrocardiographic R wave voltage (without echocardiographic evidence of increased septal or posterior wall thickness) seen in group III patients is likely related to a combination of slightly younger age and decreased body surface area, with a resultant closer proximity of the heart to the chest wall.[23] Overall, notable alterations in conduction intervals as well as P, QRS, and T wave morphology were not found. The cause of decreased exercise tolerance among group II alcoholic patients is unclear; however, previous evaluation of recently abstinent alcoholic patients (of same age and extent of ethanol abuse to those currently studied) revealed exercise duration similar to that found in group II.[24]

The present study does not assess the potential effects of recent marijuana abuse (as evidenced by positive urine tests) by three patients in group III. Exclusion of data from these subjects did not change any of the findings. Prior studies[25] indicate that the effects of chronic cannaniboid exposure on the response to orthostatic stress, ice immersion, and exercise return to pre-drug values within one day of discontinuance of drug. Moreover, unlike the increase in SBP during tilt seen in group III patients, prior studies of volunteers withdrawn from prolonged isolated exposure to delta-9-tetrahydrocannabinol have shown a decrease in SBP in response to upright posture. Though the present results suggest a primary effect of cocaine-alcohol, an additional effect of cannabis in some patients cannot be completely excluded. In addition, we did not assess the persistence of abnormalities at a later time after drug withdrawal. Therefore, based upon these initial data, further detailed studies of sinus node function and reflex blood pressure responses in asymptomatic chronic cocaine-alcohol abusers are required.

REFERENCES

1. Adams EH, Kozel NJ. Cocaine use in America: Introduction and overview. NIDA Res Monogr Ser. 1985; 61:1-7.

2. Smith DE. Cocaine-alcohol abuse: epidemiological, diagnostic and treatment considerations. J Psychoactive Drugs. 1986; 18: 117-29.

3. Regan TJ. Alcoholic cardiomyopathy. Prog Cardiovasc Dis. 1984; 27:141-52.

4. Alvaro U, Estruch R, Navarro-Lopez F, Grau JM, Mont L, Rubin E. The effects of alcoholism on skeletal and cardiac muscle. N Engl J Med. 1989; 320:409-15.

5. Tazelaar HD, Karch SB, Stephens BG, Billingham ME. Cocaine and the heart. Hum Pathol. 1987; 18:195-9.

6. Karch SB, Billingham ME. The pathology and etiology of cocaine-induced heart disease. Arch Pathol Lab Med. 1988; 112:225-30.

7. Peng S, French WJ, Pelikan CD. Direct cocaine cardiotoxicity demonstrated by endomyocardial biopsy. Arch Pathol Lab Med. 1989; 113:842-5.

8. Wiener RS, Lockhart JT, Schwartz RG. Dilated cardiomyopathy and cocaine abuse. Report of two cases. Am J Med. 1986; 81:699-701.

9. Eisenhofer G, Whiteside EA, Johnson RH. Plasma catecholamine response to change of posture in alcoholics during withdrawal and after continued abstinence from alcohol. Clin Sci 68:71-78, 1985.

10. Johnson RH, Eisenhofer G, Lambie DG. The effects of acute and chronic ingestion of ethanol on the autonomic nervous system. Drug Alcohol Depend. 1986; 18:319-28.

11. Pitts DK, Marwah J. Autonomic actions of cocaine. Can J Physiol Pharmacol. 1989; 67:1168-76.

12. St. John-Allan, Vullilet PR, Avakian EV. Effects of chronic cocaine administration on rat cardiac and splenic norepinephrine levels. Proc West Pharmacol Soc. 1989; 32:61-3.

13. Sahn DJ, DeMaria A, Kisslo J, Weyman A. Recommendations regarding quantitation in M-mode echocardiography: results of a survey of echocardiographic measurement. Circulation 1978; 58:1072-83.

14. Zar JH. Biostatistical Analysis. Englewood Cliffs, NJ: Prentice Hall, 1984:401-3.

15. Dixon WJ, Brown MB (eds). BMDP Biomedical Computer P-Series. University of California Press, 1979.

16. Foltin RW, Fischman MW. Ethanol and cocaine interactions in humans: cardiovascular consequences. Pharmacol Bichem Behav. 1989; 31: 877-83.

17. Duncan G, Johnson RH, Lambie DG, Whiteside EA. Evidence of vagal neuropathy in chronic alcoholics. Lancet 1980; 1:1053-7.

18. Dixon WR, Lau B, Chang APL, Machado J. Effect of oral self-administration of cocaine on adrenal catecholamine levels and cardiovascular parameters in the conscious rat. Proc West Pharmacol Soc. 1989; 32:231-4.

19. Avakian EV. Effect of chronic cocaine administration on adrenergic and metabolic responses to exercise. Fed Proc. 1986; 45: 1060 (abstract).

20. Tarizzo V, Rubio MC. Effects of cocaine on several adrenergic system parameters. Gen Pharmac. 1985; 16:71-4.

21. Avakian EV, Manneh VA. Cardiac responsivity to epinephrine following chronic cocaine administration. Proc West Pharmacol Soc. 1987; 30:281-4.

22. Avakian EV, Dunlap CE, Zoltoski RK, LeRoy MR. Effects of chronic cocaine administration on cardiac beta-receptor concentration in rats. Proc West Pharmacol Soc. 1987; 30:299-301.

23. Horton JD, Sherber HS, Lakatta EG. Distance correction for precordial electrocardiographic voltage in estimating left ventricular mass. Circulation 1977; 55:509-12.

24. Moskowitz RM, Parent MG, Marshall RC, Barnett CA, Errichetti AJ. Response to exercise after withdrawal from chronic alcoholism. Chest 1988; 93:1190-5.

25. Benowitz NL, Jones RT. Cardiovascular effects of prolonged delta-9-tetrahydrocannabinol ingestion. Clin Pharmacol Ther. 1975; 18:287-97.

Preventing HIV Transmission in Drug Treatment Programs: What Works?

James L. Sorensen, PhD

SUMMARY. The AIDS epidemic has dramatically affected drug treatment programs, creating both an epidemiological crisis and a psychological one. A paramount question for treatment program staff is how to prevent patients from acquiring or spreading HIV. The health belief model has been useful in generating prevention approaches, including programs that raise the threat of infection, provide alternative behaviors, and build social support. Some of these programs have been effective in changing attitudes and reducing the behaviors that put drug users at risk for acquiring or transmitting HIV. Future research will develop collaborative studies, disseminate techniques to drug treatment programs, and develop more powerful interventions for patients who continue with risky behaviors.

Drug treatment programs have been hit hard by the AIDS epidemic, both in numbers and in the psychological stresses that accompany the epidemic. In numbers, the President's Commission on the HIV epidemic estimated that there were 1.2 to 1.3 million injection drug users. However, the true number at any one time will

James L. Sorensen is Adjunct Professor of Psychiatry and Chief of Substance Abuse Services, UCSF at San Francisco General Hospital, San Francisco, CA.

This work was supported in part by the National Institutes of Mental Health and Drug Abuse (Grant P01 MH42459) and NIDA grants R01 DA04340 and R18 DA06097. The author appreciates the cooperation of the staff and patients of Substance Abuse Services, UCSF at San Francisco General Hospital.

Address comments to the author at Substance Abuse Services—Ward 92, UCSF at San Francisco General Hospital, 1001 Potrero Avenue, San Francisco, CA 94110.

never be known.[1] As to HIV-infected drug users, numbers are even less certain than number of users. There are considerable differences in geographic distribution of HIV among injection drug users, with seroprevalence rates as high as 50-60% in some northeastern cities, 15-17% in San Francisco, and below 5% of most other areas of the country. Regarding AIDS cases among injection drug users in the USA, of the 102,621 people with AIDS as of August, 1989, 27% had a history of injection drug use, including 20,619 with that as the sole risk factor and 7,173 who were men with a history of homosexual behavior as well.[2] Of the new cases in 1988, 31% had a history of injection drug use.[3] The Public Health Service has projected that there may be as many as 365,000 AIDS cases by the end of 1992, but it is cautious about projecting trends by transmission category until it can be determined whether the recent changes are one-time adjustments for previous underreporting or represent significant trends.[4]

In addition to its medical and epidemiological toll, AIDS has created a psychological crisis in drug treatment programs. As *professionals*, drug treatment providers have attended to the physical, psychological, and sociocultural stresses of HIV infection among their patients. There are greater demands on their services,[5] and program policies and practices are sometimes counterproductive.[6] In addition, as *individuals*, the people working in drug treatment programs have needed to deal with their own fear of infection and feelings of helplessness or anxiety about death. The combination of professional demands and personal helplessness creates a situation ripe for professional burnout. We could help the situation if we could provide staff in drug treatment programs with activities that would definitely slow the spread of HIV among their clients.

Drug treatment programs can be centers for AIDS prevention activities.[7] Hubbard et al.[5] point out that drug abuse treatment may have important direct and indirect effects on restricting the spread of HIV infection. It acts directly by decreasing injection drug use.[8,9,10] For this reason numerous authors have called for expanding the availability of drug abuse treatment,[11] "lowering the threshold" of treatment entry,[12] and creating low-demand treatment programs. An example of "low threshold" treatment is the work of Laporte et al.,[13] who were able to enroll 68.8% of eligible incarcerated addicts into methadone maintenance as a way to prevent them from relapsing to heroin upon their release from jail. An example of "low demand" treatment is the presentation of Yancovitz et al.,[10] which showed in a random assignment design that an "interim methadone clinic" (providing dosing plus biweekly urine toxicology and an interview) produced discontinuance of needle use far superior to a group that received urine toxicology and interview alone.

Drug treatment programs can also act indirectly as sites for reaching drug users with information about AIDS and helping them to voluntarily change the behaviors that put them at risk for acquiring or transmitting HIV. These activities will require expanding the role of drug abuse treatment professionals in the AIDS epidemic[14] and training counselors in AIDS prevention.[15]

This paper presents one fruitful theoretical basis for creating such programs (the health belief model), reviews emerging controlled AIDS prevention studies based in drug treatment programs, and suggests research for the 1990s on how to prevent the spread of HIV in drug treatment programs.

HEALTH BELIEF MODEL

Drug abuse treatment professionals can benefit from a guiding model in understanding what works to prevent HIV infection. Models help in building intervention strategies and understanding the process of change that patients go through. A good model can be a combination map (providing an overview of how the patients need to change) and itinerary (providing a series of steps in the change process). One approach that has been useful in generating preventive approaches is the health belief model.[16,17] The health belief model posits several concepts that apply especially to understanding how to prevent the spread of HIV among injection drug users.

Perceived Threat

To make changes, injection drug users must first believe that AIDS is a threat to them. Increasing the threat of AIDS can be an important first step for a prevention program. For example, in the early stages of the epidemic in San Francisco drug users knew about AIDS but did not take it personally. Studies of gay men in our city showed that a most consistent correlate of safe sexual behavior was knowing someone with AIDS.[18] However, in San Francisco at the time few drug users were diagnosed, making it unlikely that they would know someone with AIDS. We created a videotape of drug users discussing AIDS to help drug users personalize the threat.[19]

Perceived Benefit

The drug user's perception of the benefit of preventive health behaviors also influences behavior. People will avoid thinking about the problem if the threat is too great. For example, in the smoking and health area, Rogers and Mewborn[20] showed films of lung operations to smokers. The smokers did not give up cigarettes as a result, but instead stated that they did not plan to have a chest X-ray. This illustrates why fear tactics work poorly with injection drug users: They suppress and deny their apprehension. Instead, it is important to increase their belief that *there are things that work* to avoid HIV infection.

Self-efficacy

Self-efficacy refers to the belief that a person *can do* the behaviors that would protect their health (and prevent HIV infection). To increase drug users' sense of self-efficacy one might train them to be more comfortable in cleaning needles and using condoms, or role-play situations that are high-risk for needle-sharing.

Social Support

This is another key, which is so important that sometimes it is placed in opposition to the health belief model (e.g., Huang et al.[21]) rather than integrated with it. In drug abuse treatment programs several approaches have been tried to increase social support, such as self-organization of drug treatment program patients,[22] having drug users make group announcements of their intent to change, and creating a fictional character of "bleach man" to carry information to the community about how to clean syringes.

In these ways the health belief model has provided the agenda for generating AIDS prevention programs for injection drug users. Programs attempt to raise the threat of AIDS to drug users, increase their belief in the benefit of behavior change, bolster their ability to make the changes, and build social support so that the changes will endure.

WHAT IS BEING STUDIED?

Drug abuse treatment itself is being studied as a way to prevent HIV infection in injection drug users. Numerous presentations at the What Works conference discussed its direct effects in reducing drug use, e.g., Ball et al.[8] for methadone maintenance. Another question is how to maximize its indirect effect—specifically, what *to do* in drug treatment programs to prevent AIDS. Several approaches are being studied.

Small Group Interventions

Group sessions totalling 1.5 to 20 hours have been attempted in a psychoeducational format aiming to help drug users to avoid acquiring or spreading HIV infection. Such an approach fits well with the tradition of drug abuse treatment programs. The group format is efficient in that a small number of staff can work with many patients, and it can use the group setting to build social support for change. The approach has also been successful in changing the risk behaviors of gay men who were not identified as drug users.[23]

Seven controlled studies have arrived at the stage of being presented at professional meetings or published: Four were set in outpatient programs and three in residential settings (see Table 1). Additional studies are underway in NIDA-funded research projects in Massachusetts (directed by Benjamin Lewis) and the state of Washington (directed by Donald Calsyn).

As the table illustrates, most of the studies involve random assignment of subjects to small group education versus an intervention thought to be less powerful (brochures, information only, or large group interventions). They enroll relatively small numbers of subjects (between 50 and 284), which is appropriate for this stage of intervention development, where interventions should be proven to be efficacious before being implemented in a wide scale. Their followup times are very short (between immediate post-test and six

Table 1
Controlled Studies of Small-Group Education
in Drug Treatment Programs

First author, reference	Sorensen [33]	Magura [29]
Modality	Outpatient detoxification	Outpatient maintenance
Design	Randomization	Matched clinics
Comparison	6 hours versus Brochures	Education & peer group & HIV test, versus Education & peer group versus Nothing
Number of subjects	98	284
Followup	3 months	2 months
Evidence of Efficacy	Needle cleaning skills	Education: Knowledge of risk Peer: Attitude toward condoms

First author, reference	Schilling [24]	Sorensen [34]
Modality	Outpatient maintenance	Outpatient maintenance
Design	Randomization	Randomization
Comparison	Skill-building versus Information	6 hours versus Brochures
N	83	50
Followup	Post	3 months

Evidence of Efficacy	Carry condoms Discuss safe sex Intend less sex with users	Condom use skills AIDS risk knowledge Risk reduction knowledge (sex)
First author, reference	Weber [35]	Burgess [36]
Modality	Inpatient detoxification	Therapeutic community
Design	Randomization	Randomization
Comparison	Small group discussion versus Large group video & lecture	Role-play & information versus Information
Number of subjects	100	Not stated
Followup	Post	Post
Evidence of Efficacy	Approaches did not differ Pre-post improved knowledge, beliefs, & intent	Attitudes
First author, reference	Sorensen [37]	
Modality	Therapeutic community	
Design	Randomization	
Comparison	6-hours versus Brochures	
N	96	
Followup	6 months	
Evidence of Efficacy	AIDS risk knowledge Self efficacy	

months later), reflecting the fact that these studies are still underway (many have longer-term planned followups). The evidence of the efficacy of these programs varies, with most outcomes reflecting improved knowledge, attitudes, intentions, or skills rather than changed behaviors. An exception to this is the study of Schilling et al.,[24] which found that subjects in a skill-building group were more likely than information-only controls to carry condoms.

The preliminary results of these studies indicate that the group approach has promise as an AIDS prevention technique in drug treatment programs. They indicate that the approach is superior to providing information alone. However, these studies use diverse approaches and measures. The further development of the group approach will require publishing the results of the studies under-way, and then developing collaborative studies that use the most powerful aspects of these interventions in controlled, multi-site in-vestigations.

Individual Counseling

Brief individual counseling sessions have also been successful in preliminary results from one random assignment study.[25,26] In this study 1-hour counseling sessions are significantly superior to sim-ply providing brochures in increasing subjects' knowledge about reducing high risk behavior and about AIDS, their perceived sus-ceptibility to AIDS, acceptance of guidelines to reduce risk, and less likely to report unprotected sex in the month prior to follow-up.

HIV Antibody Testing and Counseling

HIV antibody testing has been controversial, yet two published studies have documented that it is acceptable to 85% of drug users in a Minnesota Clinic (0% of whom were seropositive)[27] and 99% in a Maryland drug treatment program (12% of whom were seroposi-tive).[28] Learning that one is negative for HIV antibodies is associ-ated with drug users' improved belief in their self-efficacy to avoid HIV infection and intent to decrease injection drug use.[29] It is not surprising to find that a large majority will accept HIV antibody testing in carefully protected research conditions when very few are seropositive, and that being seronegative is good news to them. However, Clark and Washburn[30] have pointed out that a variety of programmatic conditions may surround such testing, ranging from it not being available at all through being uniformly required of all patients. Further carefully controlled intervention research is needed to assess both the positive and negative effects of conducting of HIV antibody testing and counseling in drug treatment programs.

FUTURE RESEARCH

Thus far AIDS prevention research in drug treatment programs has been in the exploratory phase. Innovators have devised techniques that they thought might be effective in increasing knowledge, changing attitudes, or decreasing the behaviors that spread HIV. Clinical researchers have conducted limited experimental trials of these interventions, using a variety of study designs and outcome measures. Based on the emerging results of these studies, many of these interventions appear to be effective. What will be the directions for future AIDS prevention research in drug treatment programs? I see several developments: Consolidating efforts, disseminating techniques, and developing more powerful interventions.

Consolidation

Intervention research is moving out of a trail blazing stage and into a period of paving the roads. As the results of early studies indicate the most promising types of AIDS prevention activities, the questions will become more sophisticated: Which are the "active ingredients" of these intervention techniques? How can we better measure outcomes? Who responds best to what types of interventions? Future studies will involve collaboration across geographically different sites using common measures and prevention protocols, with the idea of developing prevention techniques that are generally regarded as effective.

Dissemination

Treatment programs will not use effective techniques automatically. Clinical leaders and staff need to learn about them, make them a high priority, practice them, and adapt them to their particular program. Future AIDS prevention programs will need to apply what is known about the dissemination of research results, trying to answer the question: "How can drug treatment staff build these interventions into their daily programs?"

More Powerful Interventions

Some people change more readily than others, and no intervention will be effective with everyone. Future research will need to identify the kinds of people who do not respond to existing prevention programs, and develop more intensive interventions for them. For example, research at the heroin detoxification clinic in which the author works found that the proportion of admissions who shared needles decreased from 55% in June 1986 to 28% in June 1988.[31] However, the proportion who shared needles with more than one partner had not changed, and those with multiple needle-sharing partners were more likely to also be using cocaine. This indicates a need to develop interventions targeted at the subset of injection drug users who use cocaine and share with multiple partners. In a similar development, a recent study found that over a third of drug users who had previously reported that they had changed their behavior because of AIDS also reported that they had not maintained AIDS risk reduction, indicating a need to find more long-lasting relapse prevention techniques for them.[32] In general, AIDS prevention research in drug treatment programs will need to identify the kinds of patients who are least likely to be affected by available interventions, and then develop techniques that will work for them.

As these techniques develop, are tested out, and the successful ones are disseminated, the professionals working in drug treatment programs will cope better with the psychological dilemmas brought on by the AIDS epidemic, because they will be taking an active part in halting the epidemic among their patients.

REFERENCES

1. Turner CF, Miller H, Moses LE, eds. AIDS: Sexual behavior and intravenous drug use. Washington, DC: National Academy Press, 1989.

2. Centers for Disease Control. HIV/AIDS surveillance report. Atlanta, GA: AIDS Program, Center for Infectious Diseases, August 1989.

3. Centers for Disease Control. AIDS weekly surveillance report. Atlanta, GA: AIDS Program, Center for Infectious Diseases, December 26, 1988.

4. United States Public Health Service. Charlottesville report: Report of the

second Public Health Service AIDS Prevention and Control Conference. Pub Health Reports. 1988; 103 (Supp. 1 [Rev.]):11.

5. Hubbard RL, Marsden ME, Cavanaugh E, Rachal JV, Ginzburg HM. Role of drug-abuse treatment in limiting the spread of AIDS. Rev Infectious Diseases. 1989; 10:377-84.

6. Mejta CL, Denton E, Krems ME, Hiatt RA. Acquired Immunodeficiency Syndrome (AIDS): A survey of substance abuse clinic directors' and counselors' perceived knowledge, attitudes, and reactions. J Drug Issues. 1988; 18:403-19.

7. Bixler RE, Palacios-Jimenez L, Springer E. AIDS prevention for substance abuse treatment programs. New York: Narcotic and Drug Research, Inc., 1987.

8. Ball JC, Lange WR, Myers CP, Friedman SR. Reducing the risk of AIDS through methadone maintenance treatment. J Health Social Behavior. 1989; 29:214-26.

9. Batki S, Sorensen J, Coates C, Gibson D. Methadone maintenance for AIDS-affected IV drug users: Treatment outcome and psychiatric factors after three months. In: LS Harris, ed. Problems of drug dependence 1988: Proceedings of the Committee on the Problems of Drug Dependence. (DHHS Pub. No. ADM 89-1605). Washington, DC: U.S. Government Printing Office, 343.

10. Yancovitz S, Des Jarlais D, Peyser N, Senie R, Drew E, Mildvan D et al. Innovative AIDS risk reduction project: Interim Methadone Clinic. Paper presented at the IV International Conference on AIDS, Stockholm, Sweden, June 1988.

11. Drucker E. AIDS and addiction in New York City. Am J Drug Alcohol Abuse. 1986; 12:165-81.

12. Young MM. Low threshold methadone treatment in the AIDS epidemic. Int Working Group on AIDS and IV Drug Use Newsletter, December 1988; 3: 16-7.

13. Laporte C, Jeffers J, Marx R, Perez J, Tardalo F, Watts L., Fontana M, Joseph H. KEEP: An effective AIDS prevention education and outreach program for heroin addicts in the New York City jails. Poster presented at the IV International Conference on AIDS, Stockholm, Sweden, June 1988.

14. Smith DE. The role of substance abuse professionals in the AIDS epidemic. Advances Alcohol Substance Abuse. 1987; 7:175-95.

15. White G, Bath J. Training substance abuse counselors to reach the intravenous drug user: The National Institute on Drug Abuse Training Workshop. Paper presented at the IV International Conference on AIDS, Stockholm, Sweden, June 1988.

16. Beck K, Frankel A. A conceptualization of threat communication and protective health behavior. Social Psychology. 1981; 44:204-17.

17. Rogers RW. A protection motivation theory of fear appeals and attitude change. J Psychology. 1975; 92:93-114.

18. McKusick L, Wiley JA, Coates TJ, Stall R, Saika G, Morin S, Charles K, Horstman W, Conant MA. Reported changes in the sexual behavior of men at risk

for AIDS, San Francisco, 1982-1984: The AIDS behavioral research project. Pub Health Reports. 1985; 100:622-8.

19. Sorensen JL, Gibson DR, Boudreaux R. Conversations about AIDS and drug abuse (videotape). San Francisco: Saccade Communications, 1988.

20. Rogers R, Mewborn C. Fear appeal and attitude change: Effects of a threat's noxiousness, probability of occurrence, and the efficacy of coping responses. J Personality Social Psychology. 1976; 34:54-61.

21. Huang KHC, Watters J, Case P. Compliance with AIDS prevention measures among intravenous drug users: Health beliefs or social/environmental factors? Paper presented at the V International Conference on AIDS, Montreal, Canada, June 1989.

22. Friedman SR, Serrano Y, Torres L, Suffian M, Nelson P, Tardalo F et al. Organizing intravenous drug users against AIDS. Poster presented at the V International Conference on AIDS, Montreal, Canada, June 1989.

23. Kelly JA, St. Lawrence JS, Hood HV, Brasfield TL. Behavioral intervention to reduce AIDS risk activities. J Consulting Clinical Psychology. 1989; 57:60-7.

24. Schilling R, El-Bassel N, Gordon K, Nichols S. Reducing HIV transmission among recovering female drug users. Paper presented at the V International Conference on AIDS, Montreal, Canada, June 1989.

25. Gibson DR, Lovelle-Drache J, Derby S, Garcia-Soto M, Sorensen JL, Melese-d'Hospital I. Brief counseling to reduce AIDS risk in IV drug users: Update. Paper presented at the V International Conference on AIDS, Montreal, Canada, June 1989.

26. Gibson DR, Wermuth L, Lovelle-Drache J, Ham J, Sorensen JL. Brief counseling to reduce AIDS risk in intravenous drug users and their sexual partners: Preliminary results. Counseling Psychology Q. 1989; 2:15-9.

27. Carlson GA, McLellan AT. The voluntary acceptance of HIV antibody screening by intravenous drug users. Public Health Rep. 1987; 102:391-4.

28. Weddington WW, Brown BS. Acceptance of HIV-antibody testing by persons seeking outpatient treatment for cocaine abuse. J Substance Abuse Treatment 1988; 5:145-9.

29. Magura S, Siddiqi Q, Shapiro JL, Grossman JI, Lipton DS et al. Outcomes of an AIDS prevention program for methadone maintenance patients. Poster presented at the V International Conference on AIDS, Montreal, Canada, June 1989.

30. Clark HW, Washburn P. AIDS antibody testing in chemical dependency treatment programs. California Society for Treatment of Alcoholism Other Drug Dependencies News, Spring 1987; 14:1-8.

31. Sorensen JL, Guydish J, Costantini M, Batki SL. Changes in needle sharing and syringe cleaning among San Francisco drug abusers. New England J Med. 1989; 320:807.

32. Des Jarlais DC, Tross S, Abdul-Quader A, Kouzzi A, Friedman SR. Intravenous drug users and maintenance of behavior change. Paper presented at the V International Conference on AIDS, Montreal, Canada, June 1989.

33. Sorensen JL, Gibson D, Heitzmann C, Calvillo A, Dumontet R, Morales E, Acampora A. Pilot trial of small group AIDS education with IV drug abusers. In: LS Harris, ed. Problems of drug dependence 1988: Proceedings of the Committee on the Problems of Drug Dependence. (DHHS Pub. No. ADM 89-1605). Washington, DC: U.S. Government Printing Office 1989:60.

34. Sorensen JL, Gibson DR, Heitzmann C, Dumontet R, London J, Morales E, Milovitch E, Lee D. AIDS prevention: Behavioral outcomes with outpatient drug abusers. Poster presented at the meeting of the American Psychological Association, New Orleans, LA, August 1989.

35. Weber J, Dengelegi L, Torquato S, Kolakathis A, Yancovitz S. The effects of AIDS education on the knowledge and attitudes towards AIDS by substance abusers in a drug detoxification setting. Poster presented at the V International AIDS Conference, Montreal, Canada, June 1989.

36. Burgess M. A study to investigate the effectiveness of role play in HIV health education groups for drug abusers. Poster presented at the V International Conference on AIDS, Montreal, Canada, June 1989.

37. Sorensen JL, Gibson DR, Heitzmann C, Dumontet R, Acampora A. AIDS prevention with drug abusers in residential treatment: Preliminary results. Paper presented at the meeting of the American Psychological Association, Atlanta, GA, August 1988.

The Tacoma Syringe Exchange

Holly Hagan, MPH
Don C. Des Jarlais, PhD
David Purchase
Terry Reid, MSW
Samuel R. Friedman, PhD

SUMMARY. For over a year, the Tacoma Syringe Exchange has been operating in spite of existing drug paraphernalia laws. One hundred fifty-four subjects have been interviewed regarding drug injection practices for the month prior to first use of the exchange and for the most recent month since using the exchange. Statistically significant reductions in mean frequency of obtaining used syringes, and in mean rate of passing on used syringes, have been reported. Mean number of times bleach was used to disinfect contaminated syringes has risen. The exchange continues to attract mainly men, median age 35, with a long history of injection. No differences have been observed in mean number of injections per month.

In order to increase utilization, new sites are planned, but expansion has been hampered by a series of legal problems. Since the exchange draws many difficult to reach individuals, it is an important location for STD screening and drug treatment recruitment. Documentation of participation patterns and barriers to exchange use, and effects upon HIV serological status are recommended.

Holly Hagan is an epidemiologist at Tacoma-Pierce County Health Department in Tacoma, WA 98408; Don C. Des Jarlais is the Deputy Director for AIDS at NDRI and Director of Research with the Chemical Dependency Institute at Beth Israel Hospital in New York; David Purchase is affiliated with Point Defiance, AIDS Projects in Tacoma, WA; Terry Reid is Section Manager of Substance Abuse Programs at Tacoma-Pierce County Health Department in Tacoma, WA; and Samuel R. Friedman is Principal Investigator at NDRI in New York.

This work was supported in part by a grant from AMFAR.

INTRODUCTION

Twenty-two percent of the United States adult cases of acquired immune deficiency syndrome (AIDS), reported through August, 1990, have been attributable to intravenous (I.V.) drug use by the case; another 52% of heterosexual AIDS cases, and 59% of pediatric cases nationwide are related to I.V. drug use.[1] The causative agent, human immunodeficiency virus (HIV), may be transmitted by contact with infected blood, semen, or vaginal secretions by the sharing of injection equipment, during sexual contact, or at birth or during pregnancy. Prevention of HIV infection among intravenous drug users, their sexual partners and offspring depends on changing injection and sexual practices. To accomplish this, AIDS prevention strategies in the U.S. have relied primarily upon education, including news media and community based education and distribution of supplies, such as condoms and disinfectant bleach.

Syringe exchange programs began in Amsterdam in 1984, as part of an extant "helping system" designed to bring drug users into treatment, and to minimize the harm to those who continue to use drugs.[2] Syringe exchanges in Amsterdam, Australia, Sweden and the United Kingdom have been opposed by groups who are concerned that provision of sterile injection equipment will increase drug use, and will do little to alter fixed injection practices. This paper will review international studies of syringe exchange, and describe the Tacoma Syringe Exchange to illustrate how methods of exchange developed abroad may be used in North America.

THE TACOMA SYRINGE EXCHANGE

Given the legal and political climate in the U.S., the establishment and sustained operation of the Tacoma and other U.S. exchanges are achievements in themselves. As has occurred in San Francisco and Seattle, the Tacoma Exchange began as an unofficial operation. A former drug counselor, D.P., became concerned about the potential for spread of HIV infection among I.V. drug users, and opened the first North American syringe exchange in 1988. This private effort facilitated the procurement of public funding and official sanction. The syringes, the furnishings and D.P.'s time were all privately donated, and he did not wait for formal approval. Thus he was able to start exchanging syringes without bureaucratic impediments. Popular support grew in response to favorable reports in the news media. The local health department began a survey of exchange participants in preparation for asking for public support of the exchange. Early on, the police chief adopted a policy that gave public health and safety needs of the community priority over those of enforcing existing laws restricting the sale of drug paraphernalia. Consequently, the police who patrol the downtown area watch for drug transactions, but do not harass people at the exchange or confiscate syringes.

Official support for the exchange has kept it operating, but has not settled the basic legal question. In May, 1989, the State Attorney General ruled that syringe exchanges violated the drug paraphernalia act. The Tacoma City Attorney withheld funding for the exchange, and the Health Department filed a lawsuit to recover support. In February, 1990, Pierce County Superior Court Judge Robert Peterson ruled that syringe exchange programs are legal on several grounds, including through the exercise of the broad powers of the health officer to circumvent an epidemic. The case was not appealed.

WHAT WORKS

This discussion of what works about the syringe exchange will examine both the operations and the impact on behavior. The Tacoma Syringe Exchange most closely resembles components of the Amsterdam helping system. It offers a variety of strategies to reduce harm to drug users attracted by the availability of clean syringes and the non-judgmental, street-based orientation of the exchange. With the general aim of diminishing the negative impacts of drug injection, these strategies include education regarding risk reduction, screening for other infections associated with unsafe injection and sexual practices, and referral to other agencies for case management.

Exchange schemes in Europe and Australia have used a variety of places for distribution, which have included the use of old commercial buildings, government offices, and mobile vans. In Australia, the most effective arrangement is a combination of fixed and mobile sites (G. Vumbaca, personal communication). In San Francisco, the Prevention Point group found that their roving exchange appealed to homeless users, and that the fixed locations were more likely to be used by persons living in hotels or apartments.[3] In Tacoma, the exchange operates out of only two locations: one in the health department's pharmacy and one on a sidewalk in downtown Tacoma (the Central Exchange). The downtown location has the advantage of being in an area with a large concentration of drug injectors, and of being able to offer counseling to exchangers. The pharmacy exchange is in the same suite of offices as the methadone treatment program, and many health department clinics. Originally, there were concerns about untoward effects on methadone clients, and about incompatibilities between exchange users and other clinic patients, but no deleterious effects have been observed.

At both locations, the same singular, essential rule applies: one clean syringe is exchanged for one used syringe. To participate, exchange users are not required to register or show evidence of recent injection. The main goal has been to bring public-health programs to those persons who are difficult to reach by traditional means. This method has minimal requirements for and accepts anonymous participation, and has been well accepted by the drug-using population. In addition to ease of use by the intended clientele, consistency is an important element in the success of the exchange. Predictable hours of operation and consistent location assure exchange users that there is a reliable supply of clean syringes. The Central Exchange was forced to move last winter, and even though the new location was only one block away, the rate of exchanges returned to normal only after several weeks.

As has been noted in Europe and Australia, the exchange can attract participants. Precise estimates of the number of exchange users are not yet available; however, from survey data and syringe counts, we estimate that approximately 500 different intravenous drug users visit the Central Exchange weekly, and an average of 50 come to the pharmacy exchange each week. Each user visits the Central Exchange approximately three times a week. Indirect users of the exchange are more difficult to estimate. Twenty-two percent of exchange users are trading syringes for other persons as well as for themselves. Anecdotal information indicates that syringes from the exchange are being sold in "shooting galleries" or elsewhere after the exchange closes.

From the beginning, the exchange has operated in conjunction with the Health Department's AIDS Outreach program. Street outreach workers are active at the site, and make contact with addicts reluctant to seek help. Staff at the exchange distribute bleach, condoms, alcohol wipes, and food; they bring warm clothes to the exchange during cold weather. In all these activities, they promote awareness of health risks, and counsel and test exchangers who elect to be tested for HIV. They also recruit active drug users into treatment programs, and offer help in obtaining services such as housing and medical care. To date, more than 150 active injectors have been recruited into methadone treatment at the downtown exchange site.

In a continuing study, one hundred fifty four subjects have been systematically selected by asking every third exchange user to take part in a brief interview for which they are paid. Subjects were asked about behavior during two referent time periods: the month prior to first use of the exchange, and the most recent month since starting to use the exchange. Injection frequency and risk behavior were calculated as frequency per month, and t-tests were used to determine statistical significance for differences in means. There is no evidence that syringe exchange is recruiting non-injectors into drug injection, or causing current injectors to inject more often. Exchange users are typically male (77%), median age 35, with a long history of drug injection (median, 15 years). This profile of exchange users resembles those in Europe and Australia.[4,5] The mean number of injections per month is practically identical before and after beginning to use the exchange (151 pre-exchange and 150 post-exchange). The assumption that the exchange would serve as a convenient location for contacting drug users reluctant to seek help is supported by the fact that 62% had not been in drug treatment during the twelve months prior to interview.

As in European and Australian studies, substantial reductions in injections that risk HIV exposure and transmission are associated with exchange use. Statistically significant reductions in mean frequency of obtaining used syringes, from 57/month to 36/month, and in mean rate of passing on used syringes, from 100/month to 65/month, have been observed. Bleach use has increased, from 71 to 106 uses per month. Participation in the exchange is associated with reduction but not with elimination of unsafe injection.

WHAT DOESN'T WORK

Many aspects of the program work very well. However, several problem areas remain. HIV testing at the exchange is not possible. The van has space for HIV counseling, but it is subject to interruptions. There are conflicts between the legal standards for informed consent and the reality that the client may not be willing to commit 45 minutes to such a session. The standards for informed consent as mandated in our state law were developed to deal with valid concerns about indiscriminate HIV testing. These standards may require modification when applied to drug injectors.

Another problem is conflicts with neighboring businesses and agencies. For example, anyone seen at the exchange is denied entrance to one of the nearby hostels for homeless persons. Distribution of large amounts of clothing and food at the exchange drew crowds, which drew drug sellers and police. Consequently, the drug trade near the exchange was discouraged, and dealers have honored this proscription.

Continued support depends on demonstration of efficacy. Evaluation of syringe exchange is complex, for several reasons. First, reliance upon self-report of sharing needles is not credible, while objective laboratory measures of sharing are awkward and expensive. Second, selection of an appropriate referent group is problematic. The sterile syringes from the exchange are dispersed throughout the local population of injectors in an uncontrolled fashion, and especially through wholesale exchangers who trade up to 100 syringes at a time. Thus, drug users designated as referents may obtain syringes that originated from the exchange. Enrolling adequate numbers of non-exchanging drug users is difficult, especially as conclusions drawn from studying "convenience samples," such as drug users who come to hepatitis B or sexually transmitted disease clinics, are confounded by the high-risk behaviors that are making these persons ill. It is difficult to separate the effects of education and counseling from that of having clean syringes, and there are no plans to segregate these efforts.

PROMISING APPROACHES

Improved access is the next major aim of the syringe exchange. Resolution of legal problems will allow its expansion. As in England and Australia, the Central Exchange is being used mainly by a narrow segment of the drug-using population, especially males with a long history of injection, who comprise the largest proportion of injectors in central Tacoma. Future efforts should focus on finding ways to enroll women, and younger persons with a shorter duration of injection. Access to these other segments of drug users will require new locations, and longer or later hours of operation and the ability to be flexible enough to change locations and hours as needed, just as drug users move about under pressure from the police, or other forces. However, much of the county is rural, which impedes penetration into networks of drug users outside the city.

Expansion in the variety of services is slowly occurring. Following the harm-reduction strategies developed in Amsterdam and the U.K., the exchange is developing into a site for public health interventions. Testing for tuberculosis has just begun at the exchange; treatment will be provided there. The exchange is well-suited for contact tracing and prophylactic treatment of sexually transmitted disease in sexual partners of drug injectors. There is potential for inclusion of a wider variety of health and social services if the essential function of the exchange is not compromised in the process.

RESEARCH RECOMMENDATIONS

Further evidence of safe injection associated with syringe exchange must be accumulated. Measurement of the effect upon rate of new HIV infections is important but difficult. As syringe exchange is brought to new injectors, it will be possible to examine its effect on transmission of hepatitis B, a disease usually acquired soon after intravenous drug use begins. In combination with other efforts designed to improve access, documentation of patterns of exchange usage would be helpful in determining how clean syringes might be distributed to more drug users. In Britain, retention rates at syringe exchanges are low; only 33% returned for five or more visits.[5] Descriptions of patterns will include average duration of use of the exchange, rates of attrition, barriers to use, and predictors of regular, continuing use of the exchange. This information will be useful in planning and adapting exchange sites to fit the needs of a more diverse drug using population. Finally, if the exchange is closed for any reason, the impact of its closure upon subsequent risk behavior will be studied.

BIBLIOGRAPHY

1. Centers for Disease Control. HIV/AIDS Surveillance Report. September, 1990.

2. Buning EC, van Brussel GHA, van Santven G. Amsterdam's drug policy and its implication for controlling needle sharing. In: Battjes RJ, Pickens RW, ed. Needle Sharing Among Intravenous Drug Abusers: National and International Perspectives, NIDA Research Monograph 80, 1988; 59-74.

3. Clark GL, Downing M, McQuie H, Gann D, Dietrich R, Case P, Haber J, Fergussen B. Street based needle exchange programs: the next step in HIV prevention, paper presented at Fifth International Conference on AIDS, Montreal, Canada, June, 1989.

4. Stimson G. Syringe exchange programmes for injecting drug users. AIDS 1989; 3:253-260.

5. van den Hoek JAR, van Haastrecht HJA, Coutinho RA. Risk reduction among intravenous drug users in Amsterdam under the influence of AIDS. AJPH, vol. 79, no. 10, 1989.

Organizing as a New Approach to AIDS Risk Reduction for Intravenous Drug Users

Meryl Sufian
Samuel R. Friedman
Richard Curtis
Alan Neaigus
Bruce Stepherson

SUMMARY. This paper looks at an innovative approach to AIDS risk reduction among intravenous drug users who are not in treatment. The new method utilizes an organizing model that involves the mobilization of drug users to promote risk reduction. This strategy targets the group as well as the individual for change.

Standard outreach techniques have had some success in achieving HIV risk reduction, particularly for behavior that reduces risk through altering drug use behavior, but still leaves many users at risk. Intravenous drug users in the Netherlands and gays in the United States have organized around HIV-related issues with some success. Preliminary evidence from New York City suggests that organizing drug users may be an effective approach for achieving significant HIV risk reduction for individual users as well as those they associate with.

Meryl Sufian, Samuel R. Friedman, Alan Neaigus and Bruce Stepherson are affiliated with Narcotic and Drug Research, Inc. Richard Curtis is affiliated with the VERA Institute of Justice.

This paper is based on a presentation given at What Works: An International Perspective On Drug Abuse Treatment and Prevention Research, October 23-25, 1989.

The research upon which this paper is based was supported by grant DA05283 from the National Institute on Drug Abuse. The views in this paper do not necessarily reflect the positions of the granting agencies or of the institutions where the authors are employed.

89

Organizing strategies and the impact these strategies have had on risk reduction behaviors are briefly presented from an organizing project in Williamsburg, Brooklyn. Finally, suggested areas for future research utilizing an organizing model are presented.

INTRODUCTION

Intravenous (IV) drug users are the second largest group at risk for AIDS in the United States. They account for 30% of all AIDS cases reported in this country.[1] Not only is this group at high risk, but their sexual partners and their children are at great risk as well. Once human immunodeficiency virus (HIV) becomes established among IV drug users in a geographic area, the drug users can become the predominant source for heterosexual and perinatal transmission. The epidemic among IV drug users initially was concentrated in the New York City metropolitan area, but it has become increasingly national and international in scope. Many IV drug users have been infected in countries such as Spain, Italy, France, and Thailand.[2]

Behavioral risk factors for HIV among IV drug users include drug injection frequency, sharing drug paraphernalia, and injecting in shooting galleries; some studies have also found sexual behaviors to be significant risk factors.[3,4,5,6,7,8,9]

Interventions like AIDS outreach and education have had some success in influencing some IV drug users to alter behaviors.[10] In New York City, Narcotic and Drug Research, Inc. (NDRI) has an AIDS Outreach and Prevention (AOP) project (funded by the NYS Division of Substance Abuse Services) that provides AIDS information, education, and referral services to IV drug users and their sexual partners on the streets and in shelters. This project has had some impact on IV drug users' risk reduction.[11] However, at least 24% of those studied are still engaging in high risk drug practices and 59% are still engaging in high risk sexual practices, as measured in follow-up interviews in 1987 and 1988.[12] Despite the fact that there has been some behavior change using a standard outreach model, there has not been enough of an impact on risk reduction. High risk behavior persists at a disturbing level which indicates that innovative strategies need to be developed in order to increase risk reduction among IV drug users. In particular, we are concerned here with reaching the large proportion of users who are not in drug treatment.

ORGANIZING

Organizing has been suggested as a technique for achieving greater risk reduction among IV drug users.[13,14] This technique is based on a model that encourages the self-organization of users around AIDS-related issues. The approach involves a group-based intervention which targets the group, and not the individual as the unit of change. Prior studies have shown that group pressure can influence drug users' risk taking and risk reduction.[15,16]

Drug users' organizations potentially have four major functions in the AIDS epidemic: (a) they can provide a political voice on issues of health care and public policy, (b) they can try to set up direct services for those already sick, (c) they can work within drug-using subcultures to convince other users to reduce their risks and to support each other in risk reduction, and (d) they can continue risk reduction efforts despite funding reductions. It is possible that drug users can parallel the efforts made by gays who have organized themselves to deal with AIDS in many cities. Gays have spoken up for their interests and as a result are able to influence policy, they have set up networks to care for the sick, and have begun a dialogue within their communities about the appropriate ways to reduce the risk of HIV transmission. This effort has led to considerable normative change and to declines in seroconversions among gays with ties to the organized gay subcultures in many places.[17,18,19] Unlike gays, however, IV drug users lack a politically influential base and network of legitimate commercial establishments. In the absence of such a base, they have lacked organizational resources for establishing AIDS organizations and have also faced repression.

On the other hand, IV drug users in the Netherlands, in a somewhat more receptive and less repressive environment, have organized to an extent. They formed *junkiebonden* (drug users' unions) in the early 1980's to attain greater tolerance and respect, as well as to receive better treatment by the government and the health care system. They began needle exchange programs as a response to a hepatitis B epidemic — which was later expanded by the government in response to AIDS — and have actively worked for risk reduction by IV drug users through word of mouth, leaflets, pamphlets and by working with local user groups to make videos as an education tool.[13,14]

In the United States, organizing of IV drug users has originated outside the drug using community. A group from the University of Minnesota is attempting to organize users in St. Paul/Minneapolis. Their strategy has been to hire a "key insider," who is a recognized member of the local IV drug user subculture, to bring other users together for group meetings. Group meetings focus on AIDS-related issues including risk reduction and on group strategies and tactics. Users are also trained to become peer outreach workers. They have found that encouraging the organization of drug users is possible, although somewhat controversial within the community. Notably, this project found that a small user organization they established was able to encourage another group to form with only minimal aid from the project staff.[20] Since this organizing effort is new, there are no data, beyond the ethnographic data, available as yet to determine how successful they will be in facilitating self-organization or influencing behavior changes.[20,21]

PROJECT INTERVENTION

In New York City, an attempt at organizing IV drug users was conducted by NDRI in collaboration with the Association for Drug Abuse Prevention and Treatment (ADAPT) to set up organizations of active drug users to strive for risk reduction. This project was the first attempt to organize users in the United States. It took place in the Williamsburg section of Brooklyn which is a neighborhood that has a high rate of reported AIDS cases and a high seroprevalence rate among IV drug users. At the beginning of the project it was not at all clear that outside organizing could indeed occur. However, based on ethnographic observations, it is clear that not only can organizing occur, but, we have found that it leads to significant risk reduction.

At the beginning of the project, two approaches, that in retrospect seem quite distinct, were used. The first approach involves an emphasis on casework in a therapeutic modality that uses group process to target individuals. The second approach is a more expansive organizing aimed at changing the subculture, which involves systematic leadership identification and development; group coordination and initiative by active drug injectors; and expansion and replication of drug user organizations. After approximately a year, the subcontractor (ADAPT) shifted its emphasis to the casework approach.

Expansive self-organization is conceived of as having several stages. Significant progress was made on the first two of these stages, and some evidence exists to suggest that the third and fourth could be accomplished with serious prospects for success. These were, first, winning trust and acceptance from local drug injectors by providing intense AIDS educational outreach and assistance in obtaining medical attention and other services; second, persuading users to use our storefront as a place to hang out for informal discussion and, relatedly, to attend weekly meetings to discuss risk reduction, organizing strategies, tactics, and events; third, systematically identifying and developing users for leadership; fourth, working with truly indigenous leadership to coordinate and initiate collective activity to try to change IV drug user subculture in ways that would promote risk reduction; and fifth, expanding and replicating drug user organizations against AIDS by indigenous leadership.

The Williamsburg organizing project included the distribution of bleach and condoms from the storefront and on the street. Anonymous HIV antibody testing and pre- and post-test counseling were initiated on a regular basis about halfway through the organizing intervention.

We have found, as a result of the organizing project, that it is possible to hold recurrent meetings of IV drug users, to involve them on an ongoing basis in assisting in concrete tasks (such as filling and distributing bleach bottles), that some are willing to spend considerable time in a location where the project is taking place, and that potential leaders can be identified and involved in a strategic process. Although we developed useful experience in these areas, we have not yet succeeded in creating a core of self-consciously involved, indigenous drug-injecting organizers, nor in determining whether and how self-sustaining and expansionistic organizations could be set up. We hope to achieve these objectives with our work in the future.

IMPACT EVALUATION

In order to assess the impact of the interventions, interviews were conducted concerning drug use and sexual behavior. The interviews were conducted twice: once at intake and once at a six month follow-up. This design allows for the analysis of behavioral changes between interviews for HIV risk related to drug use and sexual behavior. Since the organizing intervention was not an individually-focused intervention, but rather a group-focused intervention, IV drug users were recruited from the street, as well as from the groups and drop-ins to the storefront, to participate in our study. These subjects included both people who had had individual contact with the intervention and those who had not.

The following is a brief report of the impact of organizing, based on the survey data, for selected risk reduction behaviors among IV drug users. (See Tables 1, 2.) Mean monthly injections declined from 176 to 114; the percent who did not use shooting galleries in the period between interviews increased from 53% to 66%; the percent who always used new needles increased from 10% to 18%; the percent who always used condoms during sex increased from 23% to 33%; and the percent (of those who do not always use new needles) who always used bleach to decontaminate their syringe increased from 10% to 19%. Sixty percent of the subjects who reported having a drug-injecting relative, friend, or acquaintance reported teaching at least one of them how to use bleach to decontaminate injection equipment at follow-up. In addition, among those who were followed up, 47% entered treatment for their drug use and 21% were still in treatment at follow-up.

DISCUSSION

Organizing appears to be a viable strategy to promote risk reduction among IV drug users. Despite the fact that the implementation of the organizing intervention was somewhat inconsistent, it was still possible to have some success as suggested by the impact it had on behavior change. Organizing against HIV transmission appears

TABLE 1. Drug- and Sex-Related Risk Reduction Based on Organizing Model

BEHAVIOR	N	INTAKE	FOLLOWUP
Mean Monthly Drug Injections*	368	176	114
Per Cent Never Used Shooting Gallery**	323	53%	66%
Per Cent Always Used New Needles***	322	10%	18%
Per Cent Always Used Condoms***	224	23%	33%

* $p < .0001$ Paired t-test

** $p < .001$ McNemar's test

*** $p < .01$ McNemar's test

TABLE 2. Bleach Use and Teaching Bleach Use Based on Organizing Model

BEHAVIOR	N	INTAKE	FOLLOWUP
Always Use Bleach to Decontaminate Syringe*	243	10%	19%
Taught Bleach to Someone Who Shoots Up	266	----	60%

* $p < .01$ McNemar's test

to be associated with considerable risk reduction. In particular, organizing appears to have an impact on pro-active behaviors to reduce HIV transmission such as the use of bleach to decontaminate needles and/or syringes and the teaching of this risk reduction behavior to others, and the consistent use of condoms. In addition, by measuring the extent to which subjects had taught others to use bleach as a decontaminant, we were able to measure the extent to which subjects had tried to implement a more collective, group-oriented approach in which they acted on the basis of taking some degree of responsibility for other users. Thus, on the basis of the evidence we have so far, we can conclude that: (1) outside organizers can initiate the organization of IV drug users and (2) the organization of users can lead to considerable drug and sex-related risk reduction among direct participants and may extend to others whom they come into contact with.

The organizing project in New York City has provided some evidence, thus far, that organizing IV drug users is a promising approach to reducing HIV risk among IV drug users. At this time, there is a need for further research in order to gain greater knowledge about organizing drug users. Based on ethnographic observations, it is clear that organizing can indeed occur; and we see here that this leads to risk reduction. On the other hand, many questions remain — including some that are fundamental to strategic decision-making about whether organizing should be promulgated as a local or national initiative. Some of the unanswered questions that remain include: (1) Is organizing a more effective prevention strategy than standard outreach and/or can it be used to supplement outreach efforts? (2) Can organizing become self-sustaining? (3) Does organizing spread to other IV drug users in the same city? (4) Would organizing be more successful when aimed at drug users who are more socially integrated into the mainstream of society, e.g., those with a place to live or with a job?

REFERENCES

1. Centers for Disease Control. HIV/AIDS surveillance report 1989; November 1: 1-6.

2. Des Jarlais DC and Friedman SR. HIV and Intravenous Drug Use. AIDS 1988; 2 (Suppl 1): S65-S69.

3. Chaisson RE, Bacchetti P, Osmond D, Brodie B, Sande MA, Moss AR. Cocaine use and HIV infection in intravenous drug users in San Francisco. JAMA 261 1989; 4: 561-565.

4. D'Aquila RT, Peterson LR, Williams AB, William AE. Race/ethnicity as a risk factor for HIV-1 infections among Connecticut intravenous drug users. Journal of Acquired Immune Deficiency Syndromes 1989; 2: 503-513.

5. Friedman SR, Rosenblum A, Goldsmith D, Des Jarlais DC, Sufian M et al. Risk Factors for HIV-1 Infection Among Street-Recruited Intravenous Drug Users in New York City. V International Conference on AIDS, Montreal, 1989.

6. Marmor M, Des Jarlais DC, Cohen H et al. Risk Factors and Infection with Human Immunodeficiency Virus Among Intravenous Drug Abusers in New York City. AIDS 1987; 1: 39-44.

7. Page JB, Smith PC, Kane N. Shooting galleries, their proprietors, and implications for prevention of AIDS. Drugs and Society 1989.

8. Sasse H, Salmaso S, Conti S and the First Drug User Multicenter Study Group. Risk behaviors for HIV-1 infection in Italian drug users: Report from a multicenter study. Journal of Acquired Immune Deficiency Syndromes 1989; 2: 486-496.

9. Schoenbaum EE, Selwyn PA, Hartel D, Friedland GH. HIV infection in intravenous drug users in New York City: The relation of drug use and heterosexual behaviors and race/ethnicity. IV International Conference on AIDS, Stockholm, Sweden, 1988.

10. National AIDS Demonstration Research. First Annual NADR National Meeting, Rockville, MD, 1989.

11. Sufian M, Friedman SR, Neaigus A, Goldsmith D, Des Jarlais DC, De-Lena R et al., Risk Reduction After Outreach Intervention Among IV Drug Users. V International Conference on AIDS, Montreal, 1989.

12. Neaigus A, Sufian M, Friedman SR, Goldsmith D, Stepherson B, Mota P, Pascal J, Des Jarlais DC. Effects of Outreach Intervention on Risk Reduction Among Intravenous Drug Users, AIDS Education and Prevention Winter 1990; 2 (4): 253-271. In Press.

13. Friedman SR, Des Jarlais D, Sotheran JL, Garber J, Cohen H, Smith D. AIDS and self organization among intravenous drug users. International Journal of the Addictions 1987; 22 (3): 201-219.

14. Friedman SR, Casriel C. Drug users' organizations and AIDS policy. AIDS and Public Policy 1988; 3 (2): 30-36.

15. Magura S, Grossman JI, Lipton DS, Siddiqi Q, Shapiro J, Marion I, Amann K. Determinants of needle sharing among intravenous drug users. American Journal of Public Health 1989; 79: 4 (April): 459-462.

16. Abdul-Quader A, Tross S, Friedman SR, Des Jarlais DC. Street recruited intravenous drug users and sexual risk reduction in New York City. AIDS. In Press.

17. Martin JL. AIDS risk reduction recommendations and sexual behavior patterns among gay men: A multifactorial categorical approach to assessing change. Health Education Quarterly 1986; 13: 347-358.

18. Becker MH, Joseph J. AIDS and behavioral change to reduce risk: A review, AJPH 1988; 78: 394-440.

19. Coutinho RA, van Grievsen Godfried JP, Moss A. Effects of preventive efforts among homosexual men. AIDS 1989; 3 (Suppl. 1): S53-S56.

20. Carlson G, Needle R. Sponsoring addict of self-organization (Addicts Against AIDS): A case study. First Annual NADR National Meeting, Rockville, MD, 1989.

21. Alperin S, Needle R. Social network analysis: An approach for understanding intravenous drug users. First Annual NADR National Meeting, Rockville, MD, 1989.

Why Woman Partners of Drug Users Will Continue to Be at High Risk for HIV Infection

Judith B. Cohen, PhD

SUMMARY. Women infected with Human Immunodeficiency Virus (HIV) via a sexual relationship with an infected drug using partner are the second largest group of women diagnosed with AIDS in this country. Since 1983, they have been the most rapidly growing subgroup of adults with AIDS, and the increase has been even more rapid among black and hispanic women. Because they are a diverse group and are not readily identified, women partners of drug users and their needs have been unknown to or neglected by service providers and programs that could help them avoid becoming infected. More complete understanding of their characteristics and needs can help in the development of sensitive educational, preventative, and therapeutic strategies to help slow the dramatically increasing burden of AIDS-related morbidity and mortality among them and their families.

As of May 1991, at least 3,673 women in the United States diagnosed with AIDS had acquired this syndrome from a sexual relationship with an IV drug user. This is of course a conservative estimate of the real magnitude of transmission, because it only includes

Judith B. Cohen is a Research Epidemiologist in the AIDS Activities Program of the Department of Medicine at the University of California San Francisco, and the Director of the Association for Women's AIDS Research and Education (AWARE).

Support for AWARE has been provided by the California Universitywide Task Force on AIDS, the Centers for Disease Control, the National Institute on Allergy and Infectious Diseases, and the National Institute on Drug Abuse.

Send reprint requests to Dr. Judith B. Cohen, AWARE, Ward 95, San Francisco General Hospital, 995 Potrero Ave., San Francisco CA 94114.

women who were interviewed before they died, and who knew that a partner used IV drugs; it does not include the 1,275 women who were never interviewed or whose knowledge of their partner's risk behavior was limited or not shared with those who asked.[1] These AIDS statistics reflect those who were infected with HIV years earlier; indicators of current (but largely asymptomatic and unknown) HIV infection among women are even more ominous. For example, the current reports of HIV infection rates among women delivering babies in major metropolitan areas indicate that as many as one to two percent of all women bearing children in some inner city areas are HIV infected.[2] Similarly, a report on HIV infection among patients screened at New York's Bellevue Hospital outpatient clinics indicated that 2.4% of nondrug-using women were infected with HIV.[3]

The population of women who are sexual partners of drug users is a population in name only; they do not belong to a unifying social group and they have only one common characteristic, which is in their name. Although there has been limited research on who they are, the consensus among service providers, researchers, and the drug users themselves is that they are quite diverse and come from all racial, ethnic, and social class groups. Ethnographic descriptions report that some common characteristics were low perception of the risk of becoming infected with HIV, isolation, low self-esteem, with a pattern of denial and a sense of relative powerlessness about the partner's drug use.[4,5]

Some larger studies of woman partners in several cities have found that while they are of all ages, and come from all economic levels, the majority are of childbearing age, already have children, and they live near or below the poverty level.[6,7] These same studies have revealed other characteristics that are of relevance in understanding risk behavior. One has to do with drug use: while all levels are reported, the most typical pattern appears to be of some alcohol and drug use, but rarely IV drug use or use at addictive levels, with typical use of the less expensive drug alternatives than of the more expensive opiates or stimulants.

An important subgroup of women is of unknown size, because the women are so hidden, even to themselves. They are the women who are unaware of, or don't want to know about, the drug use of their partner. While "not knowing" may have done little harm, or at least have been the feasible choice among limited coping strategies in the time prior to the AIDS epidemic, it is no longer a safe option where HIV infection exists.

There is general consensus among researchers in drug use and AIDS that IV drug users have been reached by risk prevention messages about their drug use, and have adopted some practices to reduce their risk of acquiring HIV infection. But these practices are more in the nature of reducing specific drug-use injecting behavior patterns like sharing injection equipment or cleaning it with bleach.[8] However, there is also agreement that changes in drug use behavior have been much more widespread than changes in behavior to reduce sexual transmission. This is clearly the heart of the problem for reducing risk of infection among their sexual partners. Despite considerable effort directed at encouraging changes in sexual behavior, and also despite evidence that they are increasingly aware of their personal risk, drug users are still unlikely to report specific changes such as increased condom use, especially with their regular sexual partners. While similar but smaller scale educational efforts have been directed toward women partners of drug users, assessment of their relevance and efficacy must follow from a broader consideration of the women's present needs for support, treatment, and other services.

NEEDS OF WOMEN PARTNERS

From the profile information available, it is clear that many of the primary needs of woman partners are social and psychological, coming from the demands and stresses of a life where needs are greater than resources, and drug use often depletes the scarce resources available. Further, this pattern is repeated on the larger scale, in that community resources to meet these needs are also far from adequate. Specifically, there are few social and psychological services available for poor women and women of color. Additionally, cultural barriers can prevent the public admission that problems exist, and can also deter women from seeking help from the "charity" resources available. Even when the need for help is recognized, there are often competing needs, and those for children and other family members have higher priority.

Women partners of drug users also tend to have more medical service needs than average, partly because of the lifestyle circumstances already described, and partly because they are unlikely to know of or have access to the preventive services that can help them to avoid the development of major medical problems. Even though they may need help more, they tend not to seek medical services because they do not have the necessary income or insurance to be able to choose alternatives to the public health system, which requires long waits and often provides only demeaning or restricted services. Prenatal care is one example; women report lack of money most frequently as an obstacle to obtaining such care, and very few women living at or near the poverty level have any health insurance coverage.[9] For women who might choose termination of pregnancy instead, there are even fewer services for poor women. Across the United States, 50% of metropolitan counties and 91% of non-metropolitan ones have no providers of abortion services; further, only 13 states have Medicaid plans that cover abortion.[10] Finally, among those who provide pregnancy termination services, there is strong reluctance to treat those who may be HIV infected. In a 1989 report on abortion clinics in New York, 64% refused to schedule an abortion for a woman who identified herself by phone as HIV infected.[11]

Substance abuse problems are characteristic of many women partners of IV drug users, yet they are unlikely to be in drug treatment programs for several reasons. First, they tend not be injecting drug users, and most public treatment programs are for those who are addicted to injected drugs, primarily heroin. Woman users are more likely to have problems with a variety of drugs, or more recently, to use relatively inexpensive crack cocaine, and there are very few programs for polydrug or crack users. Additionally, programs for which they may be eligible are usually male-oriented, and do not admit women who are pregnant, nor do they have the flexibility in scheduling or child care provisions that would allow for participation of women with children. A recent survey of drug treatment programs in New York City found that 54% of them categorically excluded pregnant women, and 87% denied services to pregnant crack users who were recipients of Medicaid.[12]

Finally, all of the barriers to getting needs addressed that are true for women partners in general are augmented if they are also women who are from stigmatized groups such as prostitutes or lesbians. It is strange that these two groups of women, at opposite ends of the stereotyped expectations about real risk for HIV infection, should have the reputations they do. Prostitutes are often assumed to be infected and to use drugs when neither is likely to be true, while lesbians are assumed to be very unlikely to use drugs or be at risk for sexual transmission of HIV, when in fact both may be true. Members of both groups have additional obstacles to be accepted into care and treatment programs because of these stereotypes.

REACHING WOMEN AT RISK

A variety of strategies have been used to increase both knowledge and perception of HIV infection risk among women. Some preliminary evaluation provides evidence that some of the most widespread and costly efforts have not been very effective. For example, in 1988, CDC's "America Responds to AIDS" campaign addressed women at risk via sexual transmission, using billboards, public transit advertising and broadcast media transmission nationwide. However, National Health Survey interview data from the three months following the campaign indicated that fewer than one in four female respondents recalled any advertising from the campaign.[13]

While all health behavior change models include increased awareness and knowledge as necessary to the process of change, recent AIDS-related research indicates that the process of providing and personalizing information is at least as important as the content of the information provided. While materials used needs to be culturally and situationally appropriate, presenting them in a supportive peer counseling mode has been more effective than using didactic sessions led by health or social service professionals. The peer interaction process allows for recognition and discussion of mutual realities that affect perception of the extent of personal risk, and assessment of the possibilities for change. This mutual recognition allows for modelling of realistic strategies and provides role model examples that are more comfortable, appealing, and feasible than the distant, simplistic, but widely disseminated messages to "just say no."

In order to provide interactive education for women, the first challenge is locating and attracting women partners so that they can become aware of their personal risk and feel comfortable about becoming participants in prevention programs. Experience to date shows that programs based in two logical types of locations — within drug treatment programs used by their partners, and in AIDS-related programs — have in fact been unsuccessful in recruiting women partners. While systematic evaluation data are not yet available, the plausible explanation is that being expected to appear at such sites is very threatening to those who are often still having a great deal of difficulty recognizing or acknowledging their own risk, as well as the associated threats to their identity and privacy. More successful alternatives have been services offered at locations that are "OK" for women to attend, where their presence is not in itself an identification of AIDS risk, and where other needs can also be addressed.

Some prevention programs originally designed for drug users have made an effort to recruit women partners by using financial incentives. While they have reported seeing women for an initial assessment and prevention session, the rates of continuance in such programs, whether to return for test results, or to continue in a prevention followup program, have been very low, from less than ten percent to 30%.[14] In general, programs with the lowest retention rates fail to recognize that the process by which a program reaches out to women will have a major effect on success rates. The programs that demonstrate concern and support for the well-being of their participants, while at the same time recognizing the strengths they do have, will provide the necessary environment for addressing the threatening issues around drug use, HIV infection, and death. The most successful programs have been those designed and managed by women, especially by women who are peers, such as the WOMAN Inc. program in Boston and the AWARE program in San Francisco.[15]

SPECIFIC MESSAGES:
CONDOMS AND BABIES

HIV prevention programs for women partners have the same goals as all HIV prevention programs in emphasizing the need not to transmit human immunodeficiency virus. However, two aspects of prevention have been unique for women, both in their emphasis and in their probability for continued failure as prevention goals. The first is that women are seen primarily as vectors for infecting others, especially the unborn. (Those who have sex for money are also feared or blamed as potential infectors of their customers, and hence of the heterosexual population in general.) Much less concern is expressed for the risks women themselves have of becoming infected from sexual partners. For example, at the two most recent international conferences on AIDS in Stockholm and Montreal, less than ten percent of all presentations were concerned with women, and of those few, nearly all were concerned with pregnancy or prostitution.[16]

The message for prevention of transmission to or from sexual partners that is addressed to women appears to be the same as for men: abstain, be monogamous, or use condoms. For women, however, what this really means is: abstain and have no partner, get your partner to be monogamous, or convince him to use condoms if he is not. Health educators who deliver these messages to poor women and women of color should not be surprised if they are regarded as having lost all of their common sense. The first message denies normal human needs for love and support, for them and their children. The second and third contradict widespread cultural assumptions about a man's biological and sexual nature, and most unreal of all, somehow assume that any of it is under the control of women.

Efforts to increase condom promotion among women at risk have emphasized correct condom use skills, perhaps because so little is known about how to promote condom use strategies in heterosexual encounters. Intervention efforts that rely on women to introduce condoms into a sexual situation are expecting women to assume new roles in an intensely emotional and private situation. In many cultural contexts, negative connotations include presumptions of infidelity, disease, or trying to control a man's sexuality. The range of reactions from male partners can include sexual rejection, domestic violence, and termination of the relationship.[17] Clearly, there is a strong need for the development of prevention methods for women to use that are under their own control.[18]

In terms of relative risk in a sexual relationship, it is unfortunate that the probability of achieving success in introducing condom use into a sexual encounter appears to be inversely associated with the duration of the relationship. That is, the least successful rates of behavior change to reduce risk occur in prolonged relationships, in contrast to much higher reported rates of condom use in casual situations, and among those with multiple partners.[19] The most extensive use of condoms reported are among prostitutes, but like other women, they tend not to use condoms with their steady partners, even if they always use them with customers.[20,21]

Another strategy advocate to prevent the spread of HIV antenatally is to increase HIV testing of women of childbearing age. Such programs are becoming widespread in family planning and prenatal clinics, and have become close to routine in some programs. While there is no question that there is the right to know of one's HIV status, serious privacy and civil rights issues are raised when this right to know becomes transformed into a provider's right to know and a women's perceived obligation to undergo HIV testing as part of her care. The expectation is that knowing one's HIV infection status is of value, and should influence decision making about beginning or continuing a pregnancy. The evidence to date, however, is that quite the opposite is often true. Women at risk are not eager to know their HIV status, and may avoid programs that expect them to be tested. Further, knowledge of their HIV status has had little effect on decisions about pregnancy. A number of studies have concluded that HIV testing is unlikely to reduce perinatal transmission because the process that leads to reproductive decision making, or lack of it, is unaffected by the knowledge of HIV infection status.[22,23,24] The profound meaning of childbearing to women of many cultures is central to their self-worth and self-esteem. And, even before AIDS, their resistance to the "don't have babies" message was well developed.

NEEDS OF HIV INFECTED WOMEN PARTNERS

The reality is that many women learn that they are infected with HIV through indirect means, following the diagnosis of a partner or a child. Thus, they are dealing with a double impact of AIDS into their lives. Immediately, they need counseling, support, and services that recognize the extent of this shock in their daily life. Many will not know what positive findings on the HIV antibody test means. Medically, they need to know the difference between HIV infection and full-blown AIDS, and especially of the long duration that can ensue before HIV infection becomes symptomatic. They also need to understand the concept of infectiousness, both in terms of how HIV infection can be transmitted to others, and equally importantly, how it is not transmitted through casual contact or living with or hugging others. Even before this, however, they will need support through the period of shock, guilt, anger, and despair that come with this news.

For many women, the next issue is their need to fit this knowledge in among other realities, concerns, and relative priorities in their lives. Those who are already dealing with AIDS in their immediate family circle, or with already inadequate resources, even to the point of homelessness, may honestly be unable to regard this new information as being of the same level of urgency. This is not denial; when a woman needs to take care of a critically ill partner, or get the sick baby across town for help, her own infection or illness just has to wait. At this point, help from peer counseling or some case management can make life less fragmented and overwhelming. Help of greatest value provides social support and the maintenance of self-esteem, while still maintaining enough privacy that the worst irrational responses to AIDS risk do not add to the load, such as losing housing, employment, or child care. Difficult and painful choices will have to be made, even if only by default, such as whether or not to continue a pregnancy, or stay with a partner who may not be infected. Often, there are no right choices, but there can be support in making the most comfortable choice, and help in implementing it.

As HIV infection progresses, information and help will be

needed in identifying symptoms and obtaining clinical care. For women, gaining access to current treatment protocols may require major advocacy efforts, challenging rules about possible pregnancy, for example. And finally, there are those universal tasks for anyone who is dying, of taking care of personal business, and being helped to let go. For women, this process is often compounded by difficult decisions about others as well, especially for their children. Programs for women need to be able to help with plans for placement of children and may require creative legal assistance, since a mother's wishes for her children may not be what is usually recommended.

This epidemic has taught us more than we ever wanted to know about the tragedy of human suffering and early death, and about people's unfortunate panic and fear reactions to a frightening new disease. But it has also taught us much about the ability of people to care for each other. That is what women partners lives have always been about; hopefully, all who are dealing with this epidemic can learn from that caring and support, which makes all the difference in human life, and death.

REFERENCES

1. Centers for Disease Control, HIV/AIDS Surveillance Report. June 1991:8, 10.

2. Hoff R, Berardi VP, Weiblin BJ, Mahoney-Troup L, Mitchell ML, Grady GF. Seroprevalence of Human Immunodeficiency Virus among childbearing women. New Engl J Med. 1988; 318:525-530.

3. Marmor M, Krasinski K, Sanchez M et al. Sex, drugs, and HIV infection in a New York City hospital outpatient population. JAIDS, 1990 3:307-318.

4. Arguelles L, Rivero AM, Reback CJ, Corby NH. Female sex partners of IV drug users: A study of sociopsychological characteristics and needs. Presented at the V International AIDS Conference, Montreal, June 4-9, 1989.

5. Sterk CE, Friedman SR, Sufian M, Stephenson B, Des Jarlais D. Barriers to AIDS interventions among sexual partners of IV drug users. Presented at the V International AIDS Conference, Montreal, June 4-9, 1989.

6. Sowder B, Weissman G, Young P. Working with women at risk in a national AIDS prevention program. Presented at the V International AIDS Conference, Montreal, June 4-9, 1989.

7. Cohen BJ, Dorfman LE, Kelly TJ, Rila M, Garcia DR, Wofsy CB. Unsafe sexual behavior and higher risk partners: Changes over time in a prospective

study of women at risk for AIDS. Presented at the V International AIDS Conference, Montreal, June 4-9, 1989.

8. Dawson DA. AIDS knowledge and attitudes for January-March 1989: Provisional data from the National Health Interview Survey. Advance Data from the Vital and Health Statistics of the National Center for Health Statistics, No. 176. DHHS Pub. No. (PHS) 89-1250. Hyattsville MD: National Center for Health Statistics.

9. Institute of Medicine. Prenatal Care: Reaching Mothers, Reaching Infants. 1988. Washington D.C., National Academy Press.

10. Henshaw SK, Wallisch LS. The Medicaid cutoff and abortion services for the poor. Family Planning Perspectives, 1987. 16:170-180.

11. Franke KM. Discrimination against HIV positive women by abortion clinics in New York City. Presented at the V International AIDS Conference, Montreal, June 4-9, 1989.

12. Chavkin W, Driver C, Forman P. The crisis in New York City's perinatal services. N.Y. State J. Med. 1989 Nov. in press.

13. Dawson, op. cit.

14. National Institute on Drug Abuse, First Annual NADR meeting, Rockville MD. Nov. 15-18, 1989.

15. Stephens PC, Hayes BJ, Adams R, Gross M. Women working as prostitutes: Participatory/consensus-based planning for provision of mobile prevention, risk reduction, and seroprevalence activities. Presented at the V International Conference on AIDS, Montreal, June 5-9, 1989.

16. Abstracts, IV International Conference on AIDS, Stockholm, June 12-16, 1988, and V International Conference on AIDS, Montreal, June 5-9, 1989.

17. Worth D, Drucker R, Eric K et al. An ethnographic study of high risk sexual behavior in 96 women using IV heroin, cocaine, and crack in the South Bronx. Presented at the V International Conference on AIDS, Montreal, June 5-9, 1989.

18. NOVA Research Inc. Conference Proceedings: NIDA Conference on AIDS Intervention Strategies for Female Sexual Partners. Berkeley CA, March 19-22, 1989.

19. Stein ZA. HIV prevention: The need for methods women can use. AJPH 1990, 80:460-462.

20. Cohen JB, Poole L, Lyons CA et al. Sexual behavior and HIV infection risk among 354 sex industry women in a participant-based research and prevention program. Presented at the IV International Conference on AIDS, Stockholm, June 12-16, 1988.

21. Centers for Disease Control. Antibody to Human Immunodeficiency Virus in female prostitutes. Morbidity and Mortality Weekly Report, 1987 36:158-161.

22. Cohen JB, Alexander PA, Wofsy CB. Prostitutes and AIDS: Public policy issues. AIDS & Pub Policy Jnl 1988, 3:16-22.

23. Holman S, Berthaud M, Sunderland A et al. Women infected with HIV: Counseling and testing during pregnancy. Sem. in Perinatology 1989, 13:7-15.

24. Schneck M, Goode L, Connor E. Reproductive history of HIV positive women followed in a prospective study in Newark NJ. Presented at the V International Conference on AIDS, Montreal, June 4-9, 1989.

25. Wiznia A, Bueti C, Douglas C et al. Factors influencing maternal decision making regarding pregnancy outcome in HIV infected women. Presented at the V International Conference on AIDS, Montreal, June 4-9, 1989.

SELECTIVE GUIDE TO CURRENT REFERENCE SOURCES ON TOPICS DISCUSSED IN THIS ISSUE

Cocaine, AIDS, and Intravenous Drug Use

Lynn Kasner Morgan, MLS
James E. Raper, Jr., MSLS

Each issue of *Journal of Addictive Diseases* features a section offering suggestions on where to look for further information on included topics. In this issue, our intent is to guide readers to selective substantive sources of current information on cocaine, AIDS, and intravenous drug use.

Some published reference works utilize designated terminology (controlled vocabularies) which must be used to find material on topics of interest. For these, a sample of available search terms has been indicated to assist the reader in accessing appropriate sources for his/her purposes. Other reference tools use keywords or free-

---

---

x

Ms. Kasner Morgan is Assistant Professor of Medical Education, Assistant Dean for Information Resources and Systems, and Director of the Gustave L. and Janet W. Levy Library of the Mount Sinai Medical Center, Inc. Mr. Raper is Instructor in Medical Education and Assistant Director for Technical Services at Mount Sinai, One Gustave L. Levy Place, New York, NY 10029-6574.

text terms from the title of the document, the abstract, and the name of any responsible agency or conference. In searching using keywords, be sure to look under all possible synonyms to retrieve the concept in question.

An asterisk (*) appearing before a published source indicates that all or part of that source is in machine-readable form and can be accessed through an online database search. Database searching is recommended for retrieving sources of information that coordinate multiple variables, concepts, or subject areas. Most health sciences libraries offer database services which can include mediated online searching, access to locally mounted datafiles, front-end software packages, and CD-ROM technology. Searching can also be done from one's office or home with subscriptions to database services and microcomputers equipped with modems.

Of particular relevance to this issue, there are many national, state, and local organizations that provide AIDS and substance dependence information, referrals, and other services. The following agencies provide toll-free hotlines to assist both health practitioners and patients:

> Centers for Disease Control
> 1600 Clifton Road, NE
> Atlanta, Ga. 30333
> 1-800-342-2437 (1-800-342-AIDS)

> National Cancer Institute
> Cancer Information Services
> 9000 Rockville Pike
> Bethesda, Md. 20892
> 1-800-422-6237 (1-800-4CANCER)

> National Cocaine Hotline (A public service of Psychiatric
>   Institutes of America)
> P.O. Box 100
> Summit, N.J. 07902
> 1-800-262-2463 (1-800-COCAINE)

> National Institute on Drug Abuse
> P.O. Box 2345
> Rockville, Md. 20852
> 1-800-662-4357 (1-800-662-HELP)

Readers are encouraged to consult their librarians for furtlier assistance before undertaking research on a topic.

Suggestions regarding the content and organization of this section are welcome and should be sent to the authors.

1. INDEXING AND ABSTRACTING SOURCES

Place of publication, publisher, start date, frequency of publication, and brief descriptions are noted.

AIDS. Phoenix, Ariz., Oryx Press, 1985- , annual.

> See: Table of contents.

*AIDS Bibliography. Bethesda, Md., National Library of Medicine, v.1, 1988- , quarterly.

> See: Table of contents.

*Biological Abstracts (1926-) and *Biological Abstracts/RRM* (v.18, 1980-). Philadelphia, BioSciences Information Service, semimonthly. Reports on worldwide research in the life sciences.

> See: Concept headings for abstracts, such as immunology, pharmacology, psychiatry, public health, and toxicology sections.

> See: Keyword-in-context subject index.

Chemical Abstracts. Columbus, Ohio, American Chemical Society, 1907- , weekly. A key to the world's literature of chemistry and chemical engineering, including journal articles, patents, reviews, technical reports, monographs, conference proceedings, symposia, dissertations, and books.

> See: *Index Guide* for cross-referencing and indexing policies.

> See: *General Subject Index* terms, such as alcoholic beverages, drug dependence, drug-drug interactions, drug tolerance, immunodeficiency, immunosuppression, sex.

> See: Keyword subject indexes.

*Dissertation Abstracts International. Section B. The Sciences and Engineering. Ann Arbor, Mich., University Microfilms, v.30,

1969/70-, monthly. Includes author-prepared abstracts of doctoral dissertations from 500 participating institutions throughout North America and the world. A separate section contains European dissertations.

See: Keyword subject index.

Excerpta Medica. Amsterdam, The Netherlands, Excerpta Medica Foundation, 1947- , 45 subject sections. A major abstracting service covering more than 4,300 biomedical journals. The abstracts, including English summaries for non-English-language articles, appear in one or more of the published subject sections, excluding Section 37, *Drug Literature Index*, and Section 38, *Adverse Reactions Titles*, which are indexes only. Each of the sections has a comprehensive subject index. Since 1978 all the *Excerpta Medica* sections have been available for computer searching in the integrated online file, EMBASE.

Particularly relevant to the topics in this issue are Section 18, *Cardiovascular Disease and Cardiovascular Surgery*; Section 40, *Drug Dependence, Alcohol Abuse and Alcoholism*; Section 54, *AIDS*; and the sections that have addiction, alcoholism, or drug subdivisions: Section 130, *Clinical Pharmacology*; Section 30, *Pharmacology*; Section 32, *Psychiatry*; and Section 17, *Public Health, Social Medicine and Epidemiology*.

Index Medicus (includes *Bibliography of Medical Reviews*). Bethesda, Md., National Library of Medicine, 1960- , monthly, with annual cumulations. Published as author and subject indexes to more than 3,800 journals in the biomedical sciences. Subject headings are based on the controlled vocabulary or thesaurus, *Medical Subject Headings (MeSH)*. Since 1966 it has been produced from the MEDLARS database, which provides more comprehensive retrieval, including keyword access and English-language abstracts, than its printed counterparts: *Index Medicus, International Nursing Index*, and *Index to Dental Literature*. As an example of enhanced online retrieval, the check tags "female" and "male" can be coordinated with *MeSH* to limit searches by gender.

See: *MeSH* terms, such as acquired immunodeficiency syndrome; alcohol drinking; alcohol, ethyl; alcoholism; cardiology; cocaine; drug hypersensitivity; drug interactions; drug resistance; drug therapy; HIV; HIV infections; methadone; narcotics; pharmacology; rehabilitation; risk factors; sex behavior; substance abuse; substance abuse, intravenous; substance dependence; substance use disorders; toxicology; women.

Index to Scientific Reviews. Philadelphia, Institute for Scientific Information, 1974- , semiannual.

See: Permuterm keyword subject index.

See: Citation index.

*International Pharmaceutical Abstracts. Washington, D.C., American Society of Hospital Pharmacists, 1964- , semimonthly. A key to the world's literature of pharmacy.

See: IPA subject terms, such as acquired immunodeficiency syndrome, alcoholism, cocaine, dependence, drug abuse, sex.

*Psychological Abstracts. Washington, D.C., American Psychological Association, 1927- , monthly. A compilation of nonevaluative summaries of the world's literature in psychology and related disciplines.

See: Index terms, such as addiction, acquired immune deficiency syndrome, alcoholism, cocaine, drug abuse, drug addiction, drug dependency, drug interactions, drug usage, immunologic disorders.

*Public Affairs Information Service Bulletin. New York, Public Affairs Information Service, v.55, 1969- , semimonthly. An index to literature in the field of public affairs and public policy published throughout the world.

See: *PAIS* subject headings, such as acquired immunodeficiency syndrome, alcoholism, cocaine, drug abuse, drug addicts, drugs, narcotics.

Science Citation Index. Philadelphia, Institute for Scientific Information, 1961- , bimonthly.

See: Permuterm keyword subject index.

See: Citation index.

Social Planning/Policy & Development Abstracts. San Diego, Calif., Sociological Abstracts, Inc., v.6, 1984- , semiannual.

See: Thesaurus and descriptors listed under *Sociological Abstracts*.

Social Work Research and Abstracts. New York, National Association of Social Workers, v.13, 1977- , quarterly.

See: Fields of service sections, such as health and health care, substance use and abuse/alcoholism.

See: Subject index.

Sociological Abstracts. San Diego, Calif., Sociological Abstracts, Inc., 1952- , 5 times per year. A collection of nonevaluative abstracts which reflect the world's serial literature in sociology and related disciplines.

See: *Thesaurus of Sociological Indexing Terms*.

See: Descriptors such as acquired immunodeficiency syndrome, alcohol use, alcoholism, drug abuse, drug addiction, drug use, substance abuse.

Substance Abuse Index and Abstracts: A Guide to Drug, Alcohol and Tobacco Research. New York, Scientific DataLink, 1989- , annual with supplements. A multidisciplinary guide to the literature on psychoactive substance use and abuse, prevention, treatment and control.

See: Subject index.

Virology & AIDS Abstracts. Bethesda, Md., Cambridge Scientific Abstracts, v.21, 1988- , monthly.

See: Subject index.

2. CURRENT AWARENESS PUBLICATIONS

Current Contents: Clinical Medicine. Philadelphia, Institute for Scientific Information, v.15, 1987- , weekly.

> See: Keyword index.

Current Contents: Life Sciences. Philadelphia, Institute for Scientific Information, v.10, 1967- , weekly.

> See: Keyword index.

Current Contents: Social & Behavioral Sciences. Philadelphia, Institute for Scientific Information, v.6, 1974- , weekly.

> See: Keyword index.

3. BOOKS

Andrews, Theodora. *A Bibliography of Drug Abuse, Including Alcohol and Tobacco.* Littleton, Colo., Libraries Unlimited, 1977- .

Andrews, Theodora. *Guide to the Literature of Pharmacy and the Pharmaceutical Sciences.* Littleton, Colo., Libraries Unlimited, 1986.

Cocaine: An Annotated Bibliography. Jackson, Research Institute of Pharmaceutical Sciences, University of Mississippi and University Press of Mississippi, © 1988.

Medical and Health Care Books and Serials in Print: An Index to Literature in the Health Sciences. New York, R. R. Bowker Co., annual.

> See: Library of Congress subject headings, such as AIDS (disease), alcohol, alcoholics, alcoholism, cocaine, drug abuse, drugs, methadone hydrochloride, narcotic habit, rehabilitation.

National Library of Medicine Current Catalog. Bethesda, Md., National Library of Medicine, 1966- , quarterly, with annual cumulations.

> See: *MeSH* terms as noted in Section 1 under *Index Medicus.*

Page, Penny B. *Alcohol Use and Alcoholism: A Guide to the Literature*. New York, Garland Publishing, 1986.

World Health Organization Catalogue: New Books. Geneva, World Health Organization, semiannual (supplements *World Health Organization Publications* and includes periodicals).

4. U.S. GOVERNMENT PUBLICATIONS

Monthly Catalog of United States Government Publications. Washington, D.C., U.S. Government Printing Office, 1895- , monthly.

> See: Following agencies: Alcohol, Drug Abuse and Mental Health Administration; Centers for Disease Control; Food and Drug Administration; National Cancer Institute; National Institute of Mental Health; National Institute on Drug Abuse; National Institutes of Health.

> See: Subject headings, derived chiefly from the Library of Congress, such as AIDS (disease), alcohol, alcoholics, alcoholism, cocaine, drug abuse, drug habit, drug interactions, drug utilization, drug dependence, drugs, narcotics, pharmacology.

> See: Title index.

5. ONLINE BIBLIOGRAPHIC DATABASES

Only those databases which have no print counterparts are included in this section. Print sources which have online database equivalents are noted throughout this guide by the asterisk (*) which appears before the title. If you do not have direct access to these databases, consult your librarian for assistance.

AIDS ABSTRACTS (Bureau of Hygiene and Tropical Diseases, London, England).

> Use: Keywords.

AIDS KNOWLEDGE BASE (San Francisco General Hospital and the University of California, San Francisco).

Use: Keywords.

AIDSLINE (National Library of Medicine, Bethesda, Md.).

Use: Keywords.

ALCOHOL AND ALCOHOL PROBLEMS SCIENCE DATABASE: ETOH (National Institute on Alcohol Abuse and Alcoholism, Rockville, Md.).

Use: Keywords.

ALCOHOL INFORMATION FOR CLINICIANS AND EDUCATORS (Project Cork Institute, Dartmouth Medical School, Hanover, N.H.).

Use: Keywords.

ASI: AMERICAN STATISTICS INDEX (Congressional Information Services, Inc., Washington, D.C.).

Use: Keywords.

DRUG INFORMATION FULLTEXT (American Society of Hospital Pharmacists, Bethesda, Md.).

Use: Keywords.

DRUGINFO AND ALCOHOL USE AND ABUSE (Hazelden Foundation, Center City, Minn., and Drug Information Service Center, College of Pharmacy, University of Minnesota, Minneapolis, Minn.).

Use: Keywords.

FAMILY RESOURCES DATABASE (National Council on Family Relations and Inventory of Marriage and Family Literature Project, Minneapolis, Minn.).

Use: Keywords.

LEXIS (Mead Data Central, Inc., Dayton, Ohio).

Use: Keywords.

MAGAZINE INDEX (Information Access Co., Belmont, Calif.).

Use: Keywords.

MEDICAL AND PSYCHOLOGICAL PREVIEWS: MPPS (BRS Bibliographic Retrieval Services, Inc., McLean, Va.).

> Use: Keywords.

MENTAL HEALTH ABSTRACTS (IFI/Plenum Data Co., Alexandria, Va.).

> Use: Keywords.

NATIONAL NEWSPAPER INDEX (Information Access Co., Belmont, Calif.).

> Use: Keywords.

NTIS (National Technical Information Service, U.S. Dept. of Commerce, Springfield, Va.).

> Use: Keywords.

PDQ (National Library of Medicine and National Cancer Institute, Bethesda, Md.).

> Use: Cancer information, which includes acquired immune deficiency syndrome (AIDS) and other menu options.

PSYCALERT (American Psychological Association, Washington, D.C.).

> Use: Keywords.

WESTLAW (West Publishing Co., St. Paul, Minn.).

> Use: Keywords.

6. HANDBOOKS, DIRECTORIES, GRANT SOURCES, ETC.

Annual Register of Grant Support. Wilmette, Ill., National Register Pub. Co., annual.

> See: Internal medicine, medicine; pharmacology; psychiatry, psychology, mental health sections.

> See: Subject index.

*Biomedical Index to PHS-Supported Research. Bethesda, Md.,

National Institutes of Health, Division of Research Grants, annual.

> See: Subject index.

Database Directory. White Plains, N.Y., Knowledge Industry Publications in cooperation with the American Society for Information Science, annual.

> See: Subject index.

Directory of AIDS-Related Databases and Bulletin Boards. Rockville, Md., National AIDS Information Clearinghouse, Centers for Disease Control, 1989.

Directory of Online Databases (includes *Online Databases in the Medical and Life Sciences*). New York, Cuadra/Elsevier, quarterly.

> See: Subject index.

Directory of Research Grants. Phoenix, Ariz., Oryx Press, annual.

> See: Subject index terms, such as AIDS, alcoholism, drug abuse.

Encyclopedia of Associations. Detroit, Gale Research Co., annual (occasional supplements between editions).

> See: Subject index.

Encyclopedia of Information Systems and Services. 8th ed. Detroit, Gale Research Co., © 1988.

Foundation Directory. New York, The Foundation Center, biennial (updated between editions by *Foundation Directory Supplement*).

> See: Index of foundations.

> See: Index of foundations by state and city.

> See: Index of donors, trustees, and administrators.

> See: Index of fields of interest.

O'Brien, Robert and Sidney Cohen. *The Encyclopedia of Drug Abuse*. New York, Facts on File Pub., 1984.

Roper, Fred W. and Jo Anne Boorkman. *Introduction to Reference Sources in the Health Sciences*. 2nd ed. Chicago, Medical Library Association, © 1984.

The SALIS Directory: Substance Abuse Librarians and Information Specialists. Berkeley, Calif., Alcohol Research Group, Medical Research Institute of San Francisco and University of California, Berkeley, 1987-88, © 1987.

Statistics Sources. 14th ed. Detroit, Gale Research Co., 1991, © 1990.

7. JOURNAL LISTINGS

*Ulrich's International Periodicals Directory, Now Including Irregular Serials & Annuals. New York, R. R. Bowker Co., annual (updated between editions by *Ulrich's Quarterly*).

> See: Subject categories, such as drug abuse and alcoholism, medical sciences, pharmacy and pharmacology, psychology.

8. AUDIOVISUAL PROGRAMS

*National Library of Medicine Audiovisuals Catalog. Bethesda, Md., National Library of Medicine, 1977- , quarterly, with annual cumulations.

> See: *MeSH* terms as noted in Section 1 under *Index Medicus*.

Patient Education Sourcebook. [Saint Louis, Mo.], Health Sciences Communications Association, © 1985.

> See: *MeSH* terms as noted in Section 1 under *Index Medicus*.

9. GUIDES TO UPCOMING MEETINGS

Scientific Meetings. San Diego, Calif., Scientific Meetings Publications, quarterly.

> See: Subject indexes.

> See: Association listing.

World Meetings: Medicine. New York, Macmillan Pub. Co., quarterly.

> See: Keyword index.

> See: Sponsor directory and index.

World Meetings: Outside United States and Canada. New York, Macmillan Pub. Co., quarterly.

> See: Keyword index.

> See: Sponsor directory and index.

World Meetings: United States and Canada. New York, Macmillan Pub. Co., quarterly.

> See: Keyword index.

> See: Sponsor directory and index.

10. PROCEEDINGS OF MEETINGS

*Conference Papers Index. Louisville, Ky., Data Courier, v.6, 1978- , monthly.

*Directory of Published Proceedings. Series SEMT. Science/Engineering/Medicine/Technology. White Plains, N.Y., InterDok Corp., v.3, 1967- , monthly, except July-August, with annual cumulations.

*Index to Scientific and Technical Proceedings. Philadelphia, Institute for Scientific Information, 1978- , monthly with semiannual cumulations.

11. SPECIALIZED RESEARCH CENTERS

Medical Research Centres. 9th ed. Harlow, Essex, Longman, 1990.

International Research Centers Directory. 5th ed. Detroit, Gale Research Co., 1990-91, © 1990.

Research Centers Directory. 15th ed. Detroit, Gale Research Co., . 1991 (updated by *New Research Centers*).

12. SPECIAL LIBRARY COLLECTIONS

Ash, L., comp. *Subject Collections*. 6th ed. New York, R. R. Bowker Co., 1985.

Directory of Special Libraries and Information Centers. 14th ed. Detroit, Gale Research Co., 1991 (updated by *New Special Libraries*).